Thieme

Osteoporosis in Dialogue

100 Questions – 100 Answers

Johann D. Ringe

12 Figures
21 Tables

Georg Thieme Verlag
Stuttgart · New York

Prof. Dr. Johann D. Ringe
Klinikum Leverkusen
Akademisches Lehrkrankenhaus
der Universität Köln
Dhünnberg 60
51375 Leverkusen

Die Deutsche Bibliothek – CIP-Einheitsaufnahme

Ringe, Johann D.:
Osteoporosis in dialogue: 100 questions – 100 answers / Johann D. Ringe. – Stuttgart: Thieme, 2001

Translation and review of the German edition: Johann D. Ringe

Rüdigerstraße 14
70469 Stuttgart

Printed in Germany

Coverdesign: Stefan Killinger, Kornwestheim
Graphics: Ziegler + Müller, Kirchentellinsfurt
Typesetting: Ziegler + Müller, Kirchentellinsfurt
System: 3B2 (6.05)
Printing: Druckhaus Götz, Ludwigsburg
Bookbinding: F. W. Held, Rottenburg

ISBN 3-13-105861-7 (GTV)
ISBN 1-58890-074-6 (TNY)

1 2 3 4 5 6

Preface

Every day throughout the world a high number of medical doctors of different subspecialities is confronted with osteoporosis. Very often medical education and practical knowledge concerning the important diagnostic steps and the internationally accepted strategies of treatment are insufficient. Frequently diagnosis of osteoporosis is made rather hastily without the exclusion of important differential diagnoses. Knowledge about osteoporosis is generally inadequate in respect to the high and still increasing prevalence and socioeconomic burden of the disease and does not keep pace with rapid new developments.

Accordingly doctors feel often uncomfortable in daily practice when dealing with osteoporotic patients and the latter report on a lack of clear diagnostic statements and therapeutic concepts. As a consequence there are always numerous questions on all aspects of osteoporosis in the Continuing Medical Education and a need for clear answers and recommendations.

We have collected 100 "original questions" asked by colleagues after lectures on osteoporosis and worked out a *short* and a *detailed* answer for each. To keep it lifely we have not significantly changed the original phrasing of the questions. But we have put them into a systemic order according to thematic complexes such as epidemiology, risk factors, clinical symptoms, diagnosis, prevention, treatment, and special questions on senile, secondary and male osteoporosis. This structure and the index at the end will allow the interested colleague to find the topics of his own questions easily.

We do hope that the given information will be beneficial for our patients.

Leverkusen, August 2001 — Johann D. Ringe

Table of Contents

Male Osteoporosis ··· 75

Secondary and Localized Forms of Osteoporosis ··· 81

Epidemiology

1 Does osteoporosis mainly occur in industrialized countries? Are there ethnic differences?

Short answer: Osteoporosis occurs in all countries and all ethnic groups worldwide. The prevalence, however, varies considerably between different populations.

Detailed answer: The very high prevalence of osteoporosis in the western industrialized countries is mainly due to the high life expectancy (on average: women 81, men 76 years). Several risk factors of lifestyle associated with wealth may also be involved in the so-called developed countries. This means that in poorer countries the risk of osteoporosis will rise with increasing life expectancy and general wealth of the respective populations.

Certain differences, however, will remain due to genetic and sociocultural factors. Black people of African origin develop a significantly higher peak bone mass compared to white Caucasians and show lower rates of established osteoporosis in later life.

The high incidence of lactose-intolerance in the Chinese and Japanese population may increase their risk of osteoporosis. Furthermore, differences in nutrition, physical activity, and tasks in daily life for men and women may modify the prevalence of osteoporosis and the incidence of osteoporotic fractures (e.g. rural work being done mainly by women in some countries).

Table **1** Factors determining differences in the prevalence of osteoporosis in different populations

1. Mean life expectancy of men and women
2. Genetic differences contributing to the risk of osteoporosis (e.g. vitamin D-receptor gene, lactose intolerance)
3. Sociocultural differences (e.g. lifestyle, nutrition, alcohol consumption, physical activity at work or leisure, sun exposure)

2 How to explain the increase of postmenopausal osteoporosis? Is it due to extended screening or is there a true increase?

Short answer: In most countries the number of undetected and untreated patients is slowly decreasing due to an augmented awareness of the disease. But there are also data supporting the view of an absolute increase of the disease.

Detailed answer: In parallel with the considerable improvements of diagnostic methods and possibilities for prevention and therapy, the awareness of osteoporosis has increased during the past few decades. It is currently estimated, however, that only 20 – 30% of the patients are diagnosed and treated even in the so-called developed countries.

Studies from different European countries demonstrate an increase in typical osteoporosis associated fractures, which is higher than can be explained by the demographic situation of the respective country. There is no scientific explanation for this phenomenon but we suggest that the patterns of risk factors are changing (e.g. nutrition, mobility; compare with Question 1).

Worldwide activities against osteoporosis and strategies for prevention have not yet resulted in a significant reduction of the disease.

3 How frequent is osteoporosis based on densitometric assessment (not fractures)?

Short answer: Based on bone mineral density (BMD) measurements of the lumbar spine or the femoral neck in persons of age 50 years and older, the prevalence of osteoporosis is 16.5% for women and 6% for men.

Detailed answer: In different large epidemiological studies a significant inverse correlation was shown between BMD and future fracture risk. With a reduction of spinal BMD of 1 standard deviation (SD) the fracture risk increases by a factor of 2 to 5. Accordingly, the WHO fracture threshold defined as a T score value of – 2.5 SD is corresponding to a 5 – 12.5fold increased fracture risk (see Questions 20 and 21).

In a large epidemiological study by Melton et al. [1] measuring the lumbar spine BMD of at least 50-year-old women from Rochester, Minnesota, it was shown that 16.5% had values below a T score of – 2.5 SD. In a study performed by Looker et al. [2] a prevalence of 6% was found for men of the same age group when measuring BMD at the proximal femur.

The respective rates of predicted cases of osteoporosis increase by up to 30% if two or three BMD measurement sites are evaluated in each patient.

References

1 Melton LJ, Chrischilles EA, Cooper C, Lane AW, Riggs BL. Perspective. How many women have osteoporosis. J Bone Miner Res 1992; 7: 1005 – 1009

2 Looker AC, Orwoll ES, Johnston CC. Prevalence of low femoral bone density in older US adults from NHANES III. J Bone Miner Res 1997; 12: 1761 – 1768

4 How frequent is osteoporosis in men? Is there an increasing prevalence?

Short answer: The prevalence of male osteoporosis has been underestimated in the past. It may amount to 15 – 20% of all cases of osteoporosis.

Detailed answer: There is no doubt that osteoporosis occurs significantly less frequently in men than in women. The main reasons for this are the lower life expectancy of men, the higher peak bone mass (especially at cortical bone sites), and the absence of an equivalent to menopause with rapid loss of hormones in men.

A large epidemiological study performed in different European countries showed significant vertebral deformities in about 20% of men of age 50 years and older. In this study it could not be determined, however, which proportion of vertebral deformities was due to osteoporosis, trauma, or other bone diseases. Another more recent study proved that 10% of all men of the mentioned age group do have osteoporotic fractures of vertebrae.

For Germany we estimate that 9 million people are at risk for osteoporosis and 3 million do have established disease. If, from the latter, 15% were men there should be 450,000 men with clinically relevant osteoporosis in this country. Obviously, there is a high rate of undetected cases of males having osteoporosis. Very often they are treated symptomatically for chronic low-back pain.

We propose that the secular trend of increasing frequency of osteoporosis affects men and women equally. In most industrialized countries the male to female ratio of hip fractures in the elderly is about 1 : 3.

Risk Factors

5 Is excessive coffee drinking a risk factor for osteoporosis?

Short answer: Regular high intake of caffeine, corresponding to 3 – 4 cups of coffee daily, induces a negative calcium balance and thereby slightly increases the risk of osteoporosis.

Detailed answer: The literature on caffeine use and risk of osteoporosis is sparse. Probably the diuretic effect of caffeine is the main pathogenetic mechanism increasing the risk of osteoporosis. Since the tubular capacity to reabsorb calcium is limited, an increased diuresis is accompanied by an obligatory augmentation of renal calcium loss.

Data from the Framingham Study indicate that with a caffeine intake corresponding to 3 cups of coffee and more per day the risk of osteoporosis will increase. There is, however, no report on a monoetiological secondary osteoporosis due only to high caffeine intake. Similar to nicotine (see Question 7), caffeine must be considered as a co-risk factor being additive to other lifestyle risk factors. We suggest that drinking large amounts of black coffee is more detrimental than drinking "café au lait". When drinking the latter, the renal calcium loss due to caffeine may be partially compensated by the calcium supplied with the milk.

In general, coffee drinking is not a very important risk factor for osteoporosis and may become clinically relevant only in persons with excessive consumption

The well known negative effect of "Coca Cola" drinks on calcium metabolism is mainly due to its high phosphate content and only secondarily to the calciuretic effect of caffeine.

6 In the literature there are discrepant statements about alcohol: some describe positive others negative effects on calcium and bone metabolism. What is correct?

Short answer: Moderate consumption of alcohol is neither osteoprotective nor harmful to the skeleton. High alcohol intake has clear negative effects on the skeleton by direct and indirect mechanisms.

Detailed answer: There are indeed contradictory data in the literature concerning alcohol consumption and the risk of osteoporosis. This is mainly due to the fact that the amount and duration of alcohol intake are not exactly evaluated in most studies.

While in the past any alcohol consumption was regarded as potentially detrimental for the skeleton, there is evidence today that moderate intake has no negative effects nor any anabolic potency on bone tissue.

There are no prospective studies allowing a clear definition of a threshold of alcohol intake marking an increased risk. There may be varying tolerance towards alcohol between the sexes but also for individual persons. In our study on 400 men with osteoporosis, we chose a daily intake of 50 g alcohol as the threshold for increasing risk: 88 patients, i.e. 22% had this risk factor [1].

Table **2** Pathogenetic mechanisms involved in the detrimental effect of alcohol on bone

- Direct inhibition of osteoblasts, i.e. bone formation (osteocalcin declines rapidly in healthy young men after high alcohol intake)
- Malnutrition associated with regular alcohol intake (insufficient supply of protein, calcium, vitamins and trace elements)
- In established alcoholic cirrhosis there is a reduced intestinal absorption of vitamin D and calcium
- Diuretic effect of alcohol increases renal calcium loss
- Often combined risk factors: heavy drinkers often smoke, have little physical activity, irregular intake of food

Reference

1 Ringe JD, Dorst AJ, Faber H. Osteoporosis in men – Clinical assessment of 400 patients and 205 controls by risk factor analysis, densitometry, and X-ray findings. Osteologie 1997; 6: 81–86

7 Is nicotine abuse a risk factor for generalized secondary osteoporosis?

Short answer: There is some evidence that long-term nicotine abuse increases the risk of osteoporosis, especially in women.

Detailed answer: The pathogenesis of increased bone loss due to smoking is not fully understood. Different mechanisms may be involved. In women it was shown that those who smoke will have an earlier menopause, i.e. a shorter estrogen exposition of the skeleton. There is evidence in the literature that nicotine accelerates the metabolism of estrogen to inactive metabolites.

In men too, smoking is considered as a risk factor for osteoporosis, but there is no proven pathogenetic concept. Long-term heavy smoking induces arterial obliterations. A reduced blood flow in muscles and bone may deteriorate bone metabolism and favor the development of osteoporosis, mainly at the lower extremities.

As discussed for alcohol (see Question 6), the risk of smoking may overlap in frequent combinations with other risk factors, such as a lower degree of physical activity, suboptimal nutrition, caffeine, alcohol, etc.

In a study aiming at assessing potential risk factors in 500 men with osteoporosis, we identified 54 patients (11%) with high nicotine consumption. This was defined as smoking of more than 20 cigarettes per day for more than 20 years. These patients were found in the cohorts of primary or polyetiological secondary osteoporosis but there was no case with smoking as the sole risk factor for secondary osteoporosis [1]. There is no proof, however, that the detected prevalence of 11% smokers in patients with osteoporosis is higher than in the general population.

Reference

1 Ringe JD. Osteoporosis in men. In: Treatment of metabolic bone disease. Eds.: D Hosking, JD Ringe. Martin Dunitz Publ., London, 2000

8 What is the role of insufficient mobility in the pathogenesis of osteoporosis ?

Short answer: Chronic low physical activity is a very frequent cofactor in the development of most forms of osteoporosis. The well known phenomenon that complete immobility (e.g. space flight) leads to a very rapid bone loss underlines the importance of regular physical activity for skeletal integrity.

Detailed answer: It is difficult to assess the degree of physical inactivity as a risk factor. Nevertheless, there is accumulated evidence that low activity will favor osteoporosis while increased activity may contribute to prevention.

Worldwide, an increasing number of osteoporotic fractures is observed, which is higher than the expected augmentation due to the demographic changes of the respective populations. This accelerated increase in fractures is mainly explained by changes in lifestyle, one important factor being reduced mobility of people (e.g. less long distance walking or running in comparison to our ancestors).

Typical examples of inactivity or immobility with proven loss of bone are given in Table **3** (see also Questions 9 and 96).

Partial immobility due to several weeks of bed rest can already lead to a considerable loss of skeletal substance. We have observed very often that patients having been immobilized for only 4–6 weeks after fresh vertebral fractures developed multiple additional fractures thereafter during the process of mobilization. Obviously the phase of immobilization after fracture favors progressive bone loss.

Table **3** Situations and syndromes of immobility with high risk of osteoporosis

- Hemiplegia after stroke
- Weightlessness during space flight
- Osteoporosis of the lower part of the body in paraplegia (e.g. spinal cord injury, multiple sclerosis, Guillain-Barrè syndrome)

9 Mobility and sports protect against osteoporosis. Why does highly competitive sport have negative effects on bone metabolism?

Short answer: Regular moderate gymnastics or, especially, resistance training is able to maintain or increase bone substance. The negative effects of the hormonal changes induced by excessive high competition sports overcome the benefits of physical activity on bone.

Detailed answer: In a study performed on elderly people living in a nursing home we had already shown 15 years ago that a daily program of gymnastics is able to maintain bone mineral density (BMD) even in advanced age. Age-matched controls not participating in the training program showed progressive bone loss.

In the meantime these results have been confirmed by a large number of international studies. It was also shown that BMD decreases again very rapidly after the training program is stopped. From newer studies there is evidence that individually adapted resistance training is more effective in maintaining or increasing BMD than just moving with little resistance (e.g. swimming).

Young women with a very intense daily training program (e.g. preparation for Olympic games) often develop secondary amenorrhea. Estrogen deficiency is obviously a strong risk factor and significant decreases in BMD were shown in such females. The same phenomenon was demonstrated for ballet dancers.

But also men performing competitive sports on a very high level are at risk for osteoporosis due to a reduction of endogenous testosterone secretion.

10 What are the proven alimentary risk factors of osteoporosis?

Short answer: A life-long bone health-adapted diet significantly reduces the risk of established osteoporosis in later life. This diet should aim at avoiding major risk factors such as calcium and vitamin D deficiency, too high phosphate, protein and fibers.

Detailed answer: There is no doubt that a chronically insufficient calcium supply is the most important nutritional risk factor. A normal serum calcium level is essential for neuromuscular function and for numerous other metabolic processes. Calcium homeostasis has priority over the mechanical role of the skeleton, i.e. low oral calcium supply with a consequently decreasing trend of the serum calcium level will lead to an increased parathyroid hormone secretion, which will rapidly increase osteoclastic bone resorption. This means serum calcium is maintained at the expense of the skeleton.

Correspondingly, there is a secondary hyperparathyroidism in patients with gastrointestinal disorders associated with malabsorption of calcium, or in patients with vitamin D deficiency due to vitamin D-poor food and/or insufficient exposition of their skin to sunshine.

Further nutritional risk factors are listed in Table **4** according to pathophysiological mechanisms.

Furthermore different trace elements and vitamins may be important for bone health and skeletal integrity such as zinc, fluoride, boron, manganese, vitamins K and C.

Table **4** Alimentary factors influencing calcium and bone metabolism and increasing the risk of osteoporosis

Reduced intestinal calcium absorption
- Insufficient calcium intake (dairy products)
- Vitamin D insufficiency
- High phosphate intake
- High intake of oxalate, phytate and fibers (vegetarians)

Increased renal calcium loss
- High protein diet, acidosis
- High sodium chloride ingestion
- Caffeine, alcohol

Reduced synthesis of bone matrix
- Protein deficiency
- Chronic hypocaloric alimentation

11 Should diabetic patients be considered at risk for osteoporosis and its complications?

Short answer: Long-term diabetes is a risk factor for osteoporosis but there are no studies or case reports documenting secondary osteoporosis caused solely by diabetes.

Detailed answer: The pathogenetic mechanisms of the detrimental effects of diabetes on bone metabolism are still poorly understood. Intermittently occurring acidosis in diabetic patients may lead to calcium mobilization from the skeleton and increased renal calcium loss.

Diabetic microangiopathy with deterioration of blood flow in the bones is discussed as another possible pathogenetic component. This mechanism combined with diabetic polyneuropathy, however, is mainly responsible for localized osteopathy, the diabetic foot syndrome.

Earlier trials studying bone mineral density (BMD) in diabetic patients showed that lowered values were mainly found in the juvenile insulin-dependent type I diabetes. In late onset type II diabetes some patients have lowered, others elevated BMD values. Altogether diabetes is a moderate risk factor for osteopenia rarely leading to clinically relevant osteoporosis. Diabetes should be taken seriously, however, if combined with other significant risk factors for osteoporosis.

In patients with long-term, insufficiently controlled diabetes and complicating renal insufficiency, renal bone disease may develop. For prevention and treatment of this important late complication of diabetes, the most important measures are to lower serum phosphorus by intake of calcium carbonate and to increase the serum calcium level by a D-hormone analogue (e.g. alfacalcidol, 1 µg/day, see Question 63).

12 Are the parathyroid glands involved in the pathogenesis of osteoporosis?

Short answer: A secondary hyperparathyroidism does contribute to bone loss in different forms of osteoporosis. This bone loss can be prevented by calcium/vitamin D supplements or in severe cases stopped rapidly by a D-hormone analogue (e.g. alfacalcidol, 1 µg/day).

Detailed answer: Serum calcium levels in the lower normal range or hypocalcemia always stimulate the parathyroid glands. The resulting augmented secretion of parathyroid hormone (PTH) increases bone resorption and thereby bone loss and tends to normalize serum calcium. PTH also increases the activity of 1α-hydroxylase in the kidney and consequently improves the activation of vitamin D if sufficient 25-hydroxycholecalciferol is available.

A mild to moderate secondary hyperparathyroidism is very often involved in the pathogenesis of corticoid-induced and senile osteoporosis. In postmenopausal and idiopathic male osteoporosis it will develop only if an insufficient calcium/vitamin D supply is present.

Accordingly, an adequate calcium/vitamin D supply by diet plus sunshine and/or supplements is an important first step in the therapeutic strategy for most cases of osteoporosis. In patients with low normal (about 2.2 mmol/L) or already slightly reduced serum calcium (< 2.1

mmol/L) treatment with D-hormone analogues (e.g. alfacalcidol) will readily decrease PTH and increase serum calcium.

13 What is the reason that in some cases vitamin D deficiency causes rickets or osteomalacia and in others osteoporosis?

Short answer: Severe vitamin D deficiency with very low serum plasma levels causes an undermineralization of bone tissue, i.e. the clinical picture of rickets in children or osteomalacia in adults. Insufficient vitamin D supply and/or endogenous production with moderately lowered levels of 25-hydroxycholecalciferol induces secondary hyperparathyroidism, increased bone resorption, and in the long-term osteoporosis.

Detailed answer: In 1928, vitamin D (cholecalciferol) was isolated and its antirachitic potency was proven. Only about 50 years later was it shown that this vitamin has to be hydroxylated in two steps to become biologically active. Cholecalciferol is converted in the liver quantitatively to 25-hydroxycholecalciferol and thereafter in the kidney to 1,25-dihydroxycholecalciferol (= calcitriol). This second step is regulated according to the needs of the calcium/phosphate metabolism. Calcitriol is also known as D-hormone.

Depending on the degree of vitamin D deficiency in individual patients either rickets/osteomalcia or osteoporosis may develop:

1. **Severe vitamin D deficiency** (25-OH-D < 15 nmol/mL = 6 ng/mL)
   Typical laboratory findings:
   Low serum calcium level, increased alkaline phosphatase, high PTH, 25-OH-D low, 1,25-$(OH)_2$-D slightly lowered
   Bone biopsy:
   Broad, unmineralized osteoid seams
   Diagnosis:
   Rickets in children, osteomalacia in adults
2. **Vitamin D insufficiency** (25-OH-D < 30 nmol/mL = 12 ng/mL)
   Typical laboratory findings:
   Serum calcium normal, PTH moderately elevated, alkaline phosphatase normal, 25-OH-D lowered, 1,25-$(OH)_2$-D normal
   Bone biopsy:
   Reduced trabecular bone volume without increased osteoid
   Diagnosis: Osteoporosis

14 Some nutrition experts claim that milk and other protein-rich nutrients have detrimental effects on bone and may provoke osteoporosis. Is that true?

Short answer: A very protein-rich alimentation induces metabolic acidosis and increases renal calcium excretion. It is a misjudgement, however, to consider milk consumption in this context as a risk factor for osteoporosis.

Detailed answer: In states of acidosis calcium salts are mobilized from the skeleton to buffer these acid equivalents. Acidosis is a calcium robber, significantly increasing the risk of osteoporosis (cf. acidosis in diabetes, Question 11). The observation that alkalizing substances (e.g. potassium bicarbonate or citrate) are useful in the prevention of osteoporosis fits with this pathogenetic concept [1].

The suggestion that milk and milk products may have negative effects on bone due to their high protein content is not valid. Dairy products have a very high bioavailable calcium content. The high amount of calcium ingested with dairy products outweighs by far the potentially moderate increase of renal calcium excretion due to the protein content of these nutrients (Fig. **1**).

On the other hand, it is obvious that a protein-rich diet based only on meat consumption will induce the above-mentioned mechanism of acidosis and skeletal calcium loss.

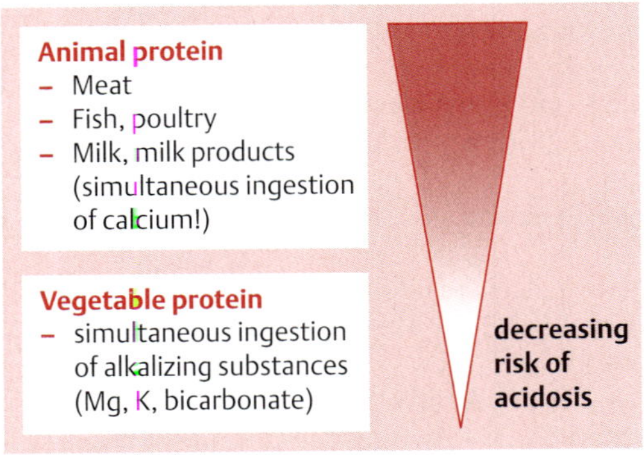

Fig. **1** Which protein should we eat?

Reference

1 Sebastian A, Harris ST, Ottaway JH, Todd KM. Improved mineral balance and skeletal metabolism in postmenopausal women treated with potassium bicarbonate. N Engl J Med 1994; 330: 1176 – 1181

Clinical Features

15 What makes osteoporosis a painful disease?

Short answer: The most frequent type of pain in osteoporosis is back pain. A distinction has to be made between acute severe pain due to fresh vertebral fractures and chronic back pain due to changes in stature together with progressive spinal deformity.

Detailed answer: From a clinical point of view osteoporosis is primarily a disease of the spine and the major clinical symptom is back pain. Pain at other skeletal sites only occurs together with fractures and will diminish with fracture healing (e.g. ribs, radius, humerus, femoral neck).

Two types of back pain can be distinguished:

1. **Acute pain syndrome:** Very severe and mostly intolerable back pain starting immediately with a first or new vertebral fracture.
   Mechanism: Fracture associated lesion of periosteum or expansion or stretching by hematoma.
2. **Chronic pain syndrome:** The chronic pain of osteoporosis is not an osseous but mainly a soft tissue and/or articular pain.
   Mechanism: Overloading of muscles and overstrain of tendons and ligaments due to progressive spinal deformity after vertebral fractures. Incongruences at small vertebral articulations.

Sometimes it is difficult to distinguish the acute pain of thoracic vertebral fractures from the pain of acute myocardial infarction, i.e. patients with osteoporosis are often seen primarily by the cardiologist.

A still unexplained question is the mechanism of the frequently observed chronic low back pain in patients with densitometric osteoporosis (lumbar spine T score < -2.5 SD) without significant vertebral deformity. Intraosseous microfractures with hematoma and microcallus formation may contribute to this pain syndrome.

16 Can a clear distinction be made between back pain due to osteoporosis and to degenerative changes of the spine if the latter are documented on X-rays?

Short answer: In most cases it is impossible to attribute back pain clearly to one or the other disorder, especially in patients with early diagnosis of osteoporosis before the first vertebral fracture.

Detailed answer: Back pain is the most frequent complaint of the locomotor system. The upright gait may contribute to the very frequent spinal problems in humans. Accordingly, back pain is one of the most frequent symptoms leading to medical consultation.

Numerous vertebral and non-vertebral disorders may provoke the symptom back pain. A thorough clinical assessment is mandatory. It is important to note that a type of pain characteristic for osteoporosis does not exist.

In patients with established osteoporosis with vertebral fractures and simultaneous degenerative changes, it is often impossible to evaluate the respective contribution to pain of the two disorders. In patients with earlier fractures and degenerative changes secondary to these "old fractures", the pain is mostly related to the latter. On the other hand a "progressive fracture", i.e. a progressive loss of height from a previously fractured vertebra, is often difficult to identify on the X-ray and could be the cause for the newly occurring pain.

The evaluation of the origin of back pain is particularly difficult in patients with stage 1 osteoporosis (BMD T score < – 2.5 SD; no vertebral fractures) and X-ray proven degenerative changes of the spine (see Question 15).

17 Clinical syndrome of established osteoporosis: What are the main problems and consequences for affected patients?

Short answer: Vertebral fractures lead to progressive deformity of the trunk and a chronic pain syndrome with consequent limitations of independence, a need for analgesics, depression, and social isolation.

Detailed answer: The main problems of patients with osteoporosis are acute back pain following fresh vertebral fractures and chronic back pain as a consequence of progressive spine and trunk deformity after one or more vertebral fractures (see Question 15).

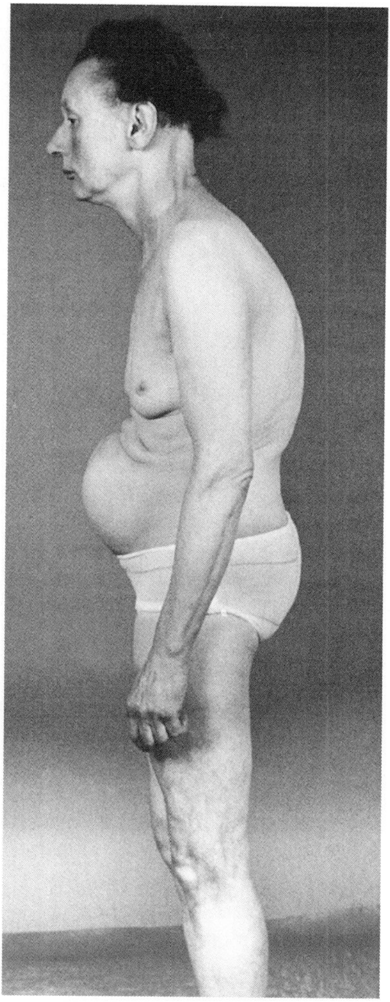

Fig. 2 Typical stature of a patient with severe osteoporosis.

Figure **2** shows the typical trunk deformity in a 64-year-old woman with severe established postmenopausal osteoporosis (stage 3) with dowager's hump, loss of height, typical skin folds, and protuberance of the abdomen.

The chronic pain syndrome and the progressive changes in stature may be followed by a number of further problems and limitations in activities and quality of daily life (Table **5**).

Table **5** Clinical problems and reduced quality of life in established osteoporosis

- Chronic pain, reduced mobility, inactivity (vicious circle for progressive osteoporosis)
- Need of help in daily life, loss of independence, nursing required
- Loneliness, social isolation, reduced sexuality, depression
- Reduced quality of life, increased mortality

18 Do patients with established osteoporosis have an increased mortality?

Short answer: Today, we have a range of very effective drugs to fight osteoporosis. The osteoporotic process can be stopped at any stage of the disease and the quality of life can be ameliorated, i.e. in general, patients with osteoporosis have a normal age-related life expectancy. Some complications of the disease, however, can augment mortality.

Detailed answer: Osteoporotic fractures, progressive spinal deformity, and chronic pain have a high impact on the quality of life but are in general not life-threatening.

Elderly patients with hip fractures, however, have a significantly increased mortality when compared to age-matched controls with similar comorbidity. The death rate within 12 months after hip fracture varies between 10 – 20% in different European countries. The most frequent causes of death are thromboembolic diseases, pneumonia, cardiac insufficiency, or simply decompensation of very instable, preexisting situations of typical geriatric multimorbidity. It must be taken into account that those who suffer hip fracture may already belong to the group of often multimorbid, frail patients.

A less frequent risk factor for increased mortality is advanced thoracic deformity due to multiple fractures with typical complications such as emphysema, cor pulmonale, and pneumonia.

Additional information: Large epidemiological studies have revealed a statistically significant correlation between BMD and mortality. Persons with low BMD have a significantly increased mortality, irrespective of underlying diseases.

Diagnosis

General Diagnostic Aspects

19 What are the most important criteria for the diagnosis of osteoporosis?

Short answer: Diagnosis of osteoporosis can be made on the basis of densitometric proof of clinically relevant generalized osteopenia (with or without fragility fractures) and after exclusion of other osteopenic osteopathies.

Detailed answer: Osteoporosis can be suspected in patients showing one or several of the following criteria:

- acute or chronic back pain,
- increased radiolucency of vertebrae on X-ray films,
- low trauma fractures in the personal history,
- low trauma fractures in their parent's history,
- loss of height,
- advanced age, and female sex.

Very often diagnosis is made solely on the basis of these criteria. This is not sufficient since every single aspect may be misleading. The most important parameter for the diagnosis of osteoporosis in women is a decrease of BMD at the lumbar spine of > 2.5 SD below peak bone mass (= T score, WHO criteria 1994). Table **6** summarizes the important steps for the diagnosis of osteoporosis.

Table **6** Criteria for the diagnosis of generalized osteoporosis

1. Proof of systemic reduction of BMD (optimal measurements at lumbar spine, hip and peripheral site.)
2. Proof or exclusion of vertebral and/or non-vertebral fractures by history and X-ray
3. Exclusion of malignant bone disease and other metabolic skeletal disorders (e.g. osteomalacia).
4. Diagnosis of primary or secondary osteoporosis by history and laboratory screening.

20 Are there recommendations for a clinical staging of osteoporosis as in other frequent diseases?

Short answer: On the basis of an internationally accepted definition of BMD thresholds for osteopenia and osteoporosis, stages of the disease have been proposed.

Detailed answer: In 1994 a publication of the WHO gave clear recommendations for BMD-related fracture thresholds in women for the first time [1].

They proposed the use of T score values of BMD, i.e. the number of standard deviations (SD) relative to peak bone mass of healthy young women of age 20 – 30 years. This definition is widely accepted today:

- T score value above – 1 SD = normal
- T score-value between – 1.0 and – 2.5 SD = osteopenia
- T score value below – 2.5 SD = osteoporosis.

This recommendation is only valid for DEXA measurements at the lumbar spine if no fractures or major degenerative changes are present or for the femoral neck. The definition is misused for other techniques, e.g. axial and peripheral QCT measurements and for different ultrasound methods. The application to other techniques increases the risk of false positive or negative results and, consequently, wrong treatment.

Taking the above-mentioned WHO thresholds together with the existence or absence of vertebral fractures, we have proposed the clinical stages of osteoporosis shown in Table **7**.

Table **7** Staging of osteoporosis based on BMD (DEXA) and vertebral fracture status

	Clinical Stage	Criteria
0	osteopenia (preclinical osteoporosis)	– lowered BMD (T score: – 1 to – 2.5 SD)
1	Osteoporosis without fractures	– reduced BMD, no fractures (T score: < – 2.5 SD)
2	Established osteoporosis (with fractures)	– reduced BMD, 1 – 3 low-trauma, vertebral fractures
3	Advanced osteoporosis	– reduced BMD, multiple vertebral fractures, often non-vertebral fractures

Reference

1 Kanis JA, Melton LJ, Christiansen C, Johnston CC, Khaltaev N. Perspective. The diagnosis of osteoporosis. J Bone Min Res 1994; 9: 1137–1141

21 What are relevant biochemical markers of bone turnover?

Short answer: We recommend the determination of one marker each for bone formation (e.g. bone specific alkaline phosphatase or osteocalcin) and one marker of bone resorption (e.g. deoxypyridinoline or NTX) if assessment of bone turnover seems to be of clinical interest in an individual patient.

Detailed answer: During recent years an increasing number of biochemical markers has been introduced reflecting either osteoblastic or osteoclastic activity, i.e. bone formation or resorption.

The accuracy and specificity of these markers are documented in large cohort studies. Especially in the large international multicenter trials with antiresorptive drugs it was shown that the decrease in markers corresponded to the subsequent increase in BMD.

In daily practice it is recommended to measure these markers not routinely in every patient but only in individual patients with a clear suspicion of osteoporosis. One marker of formation and one of resorption are sufficient (Table **8**). It has not been shown so far that proof of low, moderate, or high bone turnover in the individual patient should have any influence on the therapeutic decision (see also Question 22).

Table **8** Choice of biochemical markers for the assessment of bone turnover

Bone formation	Bone resorption
alkaline phosphatase	Hydroxyproline
bone specific alkaline phosphate (BAP)	Hydroxylysine
osteocalcin	tartrate-resistant acid phosphatase
collagen polypeptides	collagen telopeptides (NTX, CTX)

22 What is the diagnostic value of biochemical markers of bone turnover?

Short answer: The value for decision making in the individual patient is limited. In patients with antiresorptive treatment, determination of bone resorption can be used to prove compliance or non-compliance.

Detailed answer: Several experts claim that a differentiation between patients with actual low or high bone turnover is important for the therapeutic strategy. The concept is that patients with a clearly high turnover will have more benefit from antiresorptive treatment and patients with an actually low turnover might be treated with an anabolic agent (the latter is not available in most countries). The existing data are not sufficient to support this theoretically interesting concept:

1. Even modern markers of formation or resorption have a rather broad reference range, i.e. a large number of patients cannot be classified appropriately.
2. Recent fractures with abundant callus formation (i.e. high local bone resorption and formation) will result in a systemic augmentation of markers.
3. In large therapeutic studies with, e.g. bisphosphonates or fluoride, patients were never selected with either high or low bone turnover, respectively, i.e. evidence-based data are not available to prove the concept.

For the primary diagnosis in practice, an assessment of bone turnover is not necessary. There are, however, data suggesting the view that low bone density and high bone turnover are independent predictors for future fracture risk.

Indications for biochemical markers in practice could be:

- unclear, difficult cases of osteoporosis,
- resistance to therapy,
- compliance control.

23 Can osteoporosis be diagnosed from X-ray films of the spine? Or is it obligatory to do densitometry?

Short answer: In patients without vertebral fractures, diagnosis of osteoporosis is only reliable with densitometry. In patients with documented vertebral fractures, it could be sufficient just to exclude other skeletal disorders that might cause fractures.

Detailed answer: It is well known that a decrease in bone mass can be recognized only very late on spinal X-rays (about 30–40% loss). This means that osteopenia (stage 0, see Question 20) or osteoporosis without vertebral fractures (stage 1) can only be diagnosed by densitometry.

The low sensitivity of X-ray films to assess osteoporosis is due to the fact that X-rays are polychromatic (polyenergetic), i.e. the absorption of radiation by bone tissue depends not only on bone density but also on the energy of the individual photons. Further disturbing factors can be differences in X-ray film quality, exposure, and development.

In patients with established osteoporosis, the diagnosis can, of course, be made without densitometry. Low-trauma fractures *per se* document the fragility of bones. Fractures due to malignancy or other metabolic bone diseases have to be excluded, however.

If densitometry is available it should be performed also in established osteoporosis. The risk of further fractures can be estimated and densitometry can be used as a parameter of treatment control/treatment response.

Special advice: Normal bone density at the lumbar spine in patients with fractures at the thoracic spine may be an indicator for non-osteoporotic fractures necessitating further diagnostic measures.

24 Is there a screening method for osteoporosis which is easy to handle and inexpensive?

Short answer: Different laboratory tests (gene polymorphism, biochemical markers of bone turnover) have been praised as screening methods for osteoporosis. Up to now no sufficiently sensitive laboratory test is available. Today BMD determination is a suitable screening tool. Risk factor assessment by means of questionnaires can be used for prescreening.

Detailed answer: Studies on large patient groups have demonstrated an unequivocal correlation between BMD and future fracture risk. BMD is predictive for the individual patient. Biochemical markers have been shown to be a second independent predictor. The predictive value, however, is lower for the individual patient (see Question 22) and the determination of two markers is more expensive than a BMD measurement at the lumbar spine and hip by DEXA.

Some years ago the determination of vitamin D receptor gene status was suggested as a screening method. The positive results of the first published study from Australia could not be confirmed by other groups.

Conclusion: Today BMD measurement (e.g. DEXA at lumbar spine and total hip) is the most relevant and rather low-priced screening method for osteoporosis.

Risk factor assessment: Risk factor assessment by standardized questionnaires is, of course, an interesting and very cheap approach. There are, however, only few strong risk factors (Table **9**) and a large number of potentially contributing risk factor, which are often difficult to assess (e.g. smoking, alcohol, caffeine, low-calcium diet, inactivity). The value of risk factor assessment depends on the quality of the used questionnaire. It can be recommended as a prescreening measure before BMD measurement.

Table **9** Strong independent risk factors for osteoporosis

- Advanced age
- Low body mass index
- High bone turnover
- Prevalent vertebral fractures
- Prevalent non-vertebral fractures
- Fractures in the next relationship

25 Should bone mineral measurements be used for screening? And at what age?

Short answer: A general screening for osteoporosis by bone densitometry would be very useful and effective but cannot be realized in most countries for economic reasons.

Detailed answer: Taking into account the high prevalence of osteoporosis (on average 30% of postmenopausal women), a large number of cases could be identified by densitometric screening. Preventive measures, such as changes of risk factors of individual life style, could be started and preventive treatments with rather cheap substances (calcium, vitamin D, estrogens) could be initiated. For healthcare systems, the very high economic burden of vertebral and hip fractures could be reduced. There are sufficient data supporting the view that the cost-utility ratio of BMD screening might be unequivocally higher than for several other approved screening approaches (e.g. mammography).

For women, screening should be performed at the age of 50 years, i.e. the average time of menopause. But also screening at an age of about 30 years (time of peak bone mass) would be of high interest. Even a screening for men could be justified since the estimated prevalence of male cases of osteoporosis is 10–15% in men aged 50 years and over.

Further information: Very often in daily practice we see patients with a false diagnosis of osteoporosis made only from X-rays or insufficient techniques of bone mineral measurement. Expensive drug treatments can be stopped in these patients, i.e. a correct BMD determination (e.g. by DEXA) may even help to reduce healthcare expenses.

26 Is ultrasound measurement of skin thickness a reliable method for the early diagnosis of osteoporosis?

Short answer: Measurement of skin thickness is unsuitable for a risk assessment of osteoporosis.

Detailed answer: About 30 years ago measurements of skinfold thickness of the upper arm were performed to study the correlation with osteoporosis.

When more precise measurements of skin thickness using ultrasound became available some experts suggested this parameter as a surrogate for bone density.

Our group and other authors have clearly shown that there is only a very weak correlation between skin thickness and the degree of osteoporosis, probably due to the independent correlation of age with both parameters. Measurement of skin thickness is inferior to all techniques of densitometry using X-rays, isotope radiation, or ultrasound on the bone existing today.

Slovently said: "The predictive value of skin thickness for the assessment of osteoporosis is no better than the count of grey hair". In large cohorts there will always be a small correlation but for the individual case the result of skin measurement may be extremely misleading (e.g. in long-term glucocorticoid therapy a loss in skin thickness may develop much earlier than bone loss).

27 Can you recommend the evaluation of the trabecular bone pattern of the proximal femur (Singh Index) as a cheap alternative to bone densitometry?

Short answer: All methods with quantitative measurement of bone mineral content or bone stiffness are unequivocally superior to the comparative qualitative evaluation of trabecular bone architecture at the proximal femur according to Singh. If bone densitometry is not available, the Singh Index allows a rough assessment of the degree of osteoporosis.

Detailed answer: For evaluation of osteoporosis according to Singh, X-rays of a previously not fractured proximal femur are compared to schematic pictures (Fig. **3**) representing 7 different degrees from normal to severe osteoporosis. This method was described before SPA, the first densitometric technique, became available.

The results may be improved by the quality of the X-ray pictures and the experience of the observer. In poor countries or regions where modern tools for densitometry are not available, the Singh index can be recommended for a rough orientation of the skeletal status. It may be better than a qualitative estimation of radiolucency on spinal X-rays.

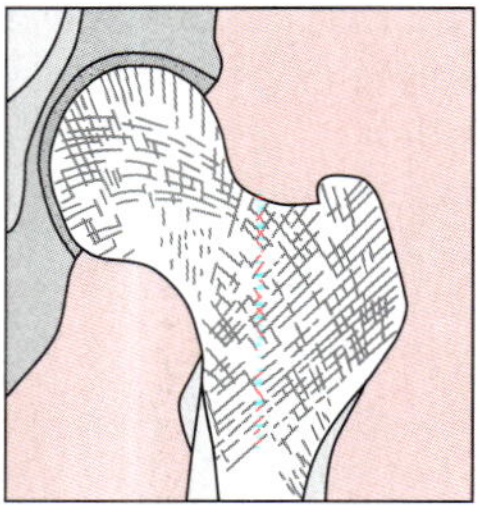

grade **7** normal

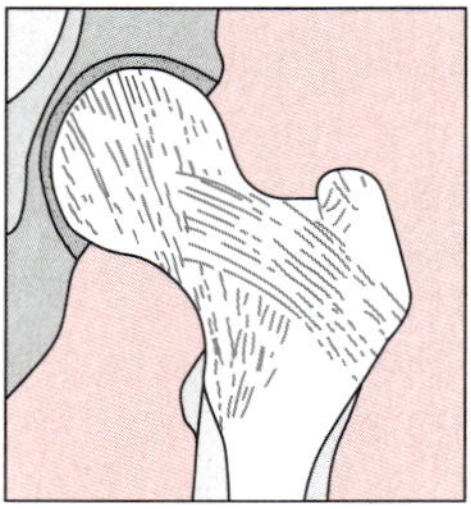

grade **6** normal

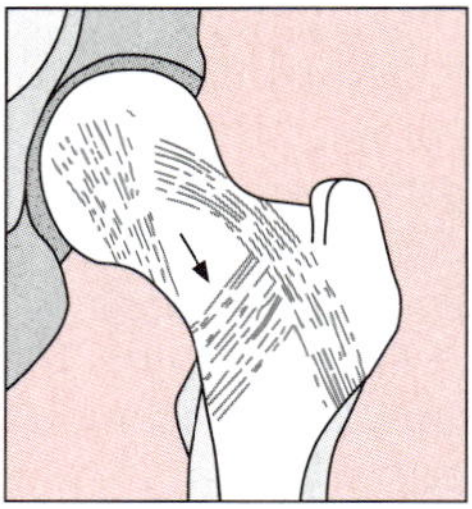

grade **5** normal

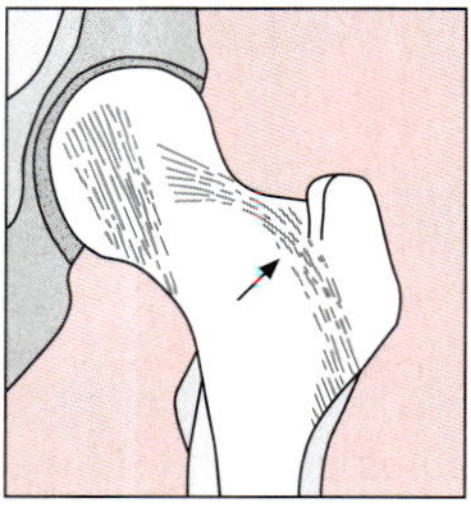

grade **4** osteoporosis

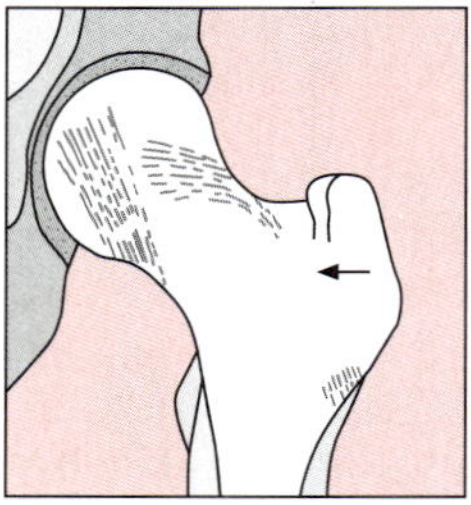

grade **3** osteoporosis

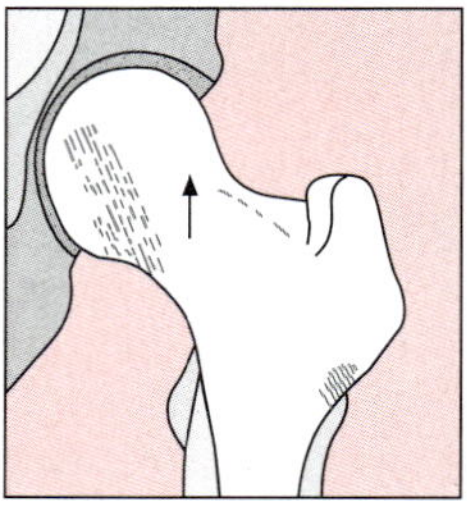

grade **2** osteoporosis

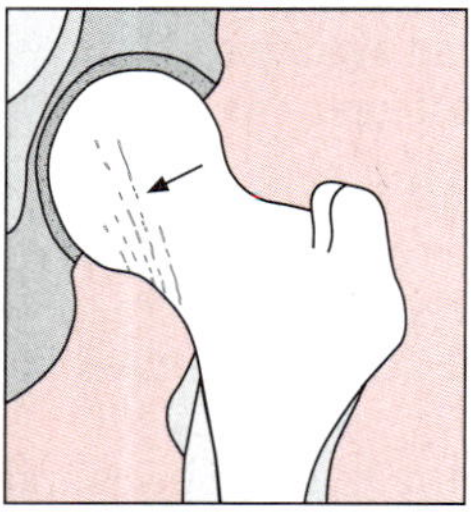

grade **1** osteoporosis

Fig. **3** Different degrees of loss of trabecular bone architecture (osteopenia) at the proximal femur from normal to severe osteoporosis (according to Singh).

Densitometry

28 How reliable are the most commonly used densitometric methods?

Short answer: The diagnostic value of densitometry depends mainly on the adopted measuring technique but also on the examined skeletal area, the methodological experience with the method, patient positioning, and the interpretation of the data.

The result describes a statistical risk for fracture but is not the diagnosis of a disease.

Detailed answer: All quantitative radiological and sonographic methods for the assessment of bone strength allow an estimation of the future fracture risk, provided that they are performed and interpreted correctly.

From our experience, the diagnostic value increases from the various ultrasound techniques, to peripheral QCT, axial QCT, through to DEXA. The latter is today regarded as the gold standard and is required for all large multicenter drug studies aiming at the approval of new substances for treatment. Their reliability can be improved by measuring two sites, e.g. lumbar spine and femoral neck or total hip. This is true for first measurements for assessing fracture risk and for follow-up during prevention or therapy. Long-term experience with the method and knowledge of potential interfering factors is crucial for valid results (e.g. with lumbar spine DEXA: vertebral fractures, degenerative changes, aortic calcification).

Repeated measurements should always be done with the same technique and if possible even with the same machine.

29 How should we interpret those cases with very divergent findings at the lumbar spine and femoral neck?

Short answer: The two most frequent underlying situations with discrepant BMD results are:

1. Dominant osteoporosis at the axial skeleton with only mild osteopenia at the hip region in women with early postmenopausal osteoporosis.

2. Significant osteopenia at the hip with falsely high values at the lumbar spine due to severe degenerative changes (osteochondrosis, spondylosis deformans).

Detailed answer: Concordant densitometric findings at the lumbar spine and proximal femur are observed in only 50–60% of patients. Divergent results in both directions are rather frequent.

Osteoporosis is a systemic, generalized bone disease. The pattern of osteopenia at the skeleton is symmetrical but not always homogeneous. Especially in patients with early postmenopausal osteoporosis, the axial skeleton (spine) will be predominantly involved due to primary loss of trabecular bone. In such cases the femur neck often shows only moderate osteopenia and at the radius shaft (containing 98% cortical bone) normal values may be found.

The opposite, rather high density at the lumbar spine and low values at the hip, is mostly due to advanced degenerative changes with increasing age (for further factors causing discrepant results see Question 33).

Very high BMD values at individual lumbar vertebrae may be due to osteoplastic metastases.

30 In men osteoporosis is frequently underestimated when measuring the lumbar spine. What is the reason for this?

Short answer: In men there is a significantly higher prevalence of degenerative changes at the vertebral bodies and the small intervertebral joints.

Detailed answer: Chronic disk problems with loss of disk height are always combined with sclerosis of adjacent vertebral endplates (osteochondrosis). A secondary development of osteophytes is very common (spondylosis deformans). These changes always lead to local hypermineralization.

With the anterior-posterior measuring procedure of DEXA, these hyperostotic spots are within the measuring area augmenting BMD values. These findings are more frequent in men than in women, especially in professions with strong mechanical loading or stress.

31 How often or at what intervals should bone density be measured?

Short answer: During treatment of established osteoporosis, controls of BMD should be performed in general at 12-month intervals. BMD measurements every 2 years may be suitable during preventive treatment or early therapy for stage 1 osteoporosis.

Detailed answer: Theoretically the intervals of densitometric controls should be adapted to the precision of the method used, the dynamics of the osteoporotic process, and the expected efficacy of the adopted therapeutic regimen.

For most methods intervals of less than 2 years would turn out to be unnecessary. Nevertheless, we recommend yearly controls in established osteoporosis. The methods are safe and inexpensive and important for long-term compliance.

After one year, in general, only a trend and not significant changes can be demonstrated (e.g. 2 – 3% increase of lumbar spine BMD).

There are some exceptions:

- In patients with rapidly progressive osteoporosis due to high doses of corticosteroids or after organ transplantation.
- Six monthly controls may be of scientific interest during clinical trials with new drugs.

32 Changes of BMD after one year – what is realistic and what is not plausible?

Short answer: If very high changing rates of 10–25% per year are measured one has to search for possible disturbing factors at the respective skeletal site.

Detailed answer: The usual change of BMD varies depending on the method and measuring site. Using DEXA as the gold standard, annual losses of 1 – 3% are realistic in untreated postmenopausal women. In patients on high-dose corticosteroids a 6 – 10% loss per year may occur.

In patients under antiosteoporotic therapy the prospective increase of BMD depends again on the method and measuring site as well as on the adopted drug or combined therapeutic strategy. The lack or intensity of a concomitant training program may significantly modify the outcome. The usual rates of increase with calcium/vitamin D, HRT, raloxifen, calcitonin, alfacalcidol are in the range of 1 – 4% per year at the lumbar spine. With oral bisphosphonate treatment (etidronate, alendronate, risedronate, ibandronate) it may be the same or somewhat higher with the more potent bisphosphonates.

Much higher positive or negative changes are suspicious. One must check whether the region of interest was taken correctly or if there are new fractures at the measuring site. A fresh crush fracture may provoke a very high increase in BMD. For other factors possibly influencing BMD, see Question 33.

Important: It has to be taken into consideration that the percentage of increase depends on the initial value. The same rate of increase in g/cm^2 will give a higher percentage of increase in patients with very low BMD.

33 What are the most frequent sources of error when using the DEXA technique?

Short answer: Different changes in the physical density of the measuring site not associated with changes of osteoporosis can modify the values and lead to false positive or negative results.

Detailed answer: The DEXA technique is based on absorptiometry, i.e. the weakening of a well defined radiation beam during penetration of the body. This weakening is mainly influenced by the calcium content in the pathway of the beam, calcium being the element with the highest atomic number in human tissues. Table **10** lists factors that may change the local absorption of radiation, thereby influencing the results of the BMD measurement. It becomes evident that there is a lower risk of disturbing factors at the proximal femur, i.e. the hip is a safer measuring site.

Table **10** Disturbing factors when measuring BMD at the lumbar spine with DEXA

- advanced aortic sclerosis and calcification
- extraosseous calcification (e.g. myositis ossificans)
- osteochondrosis, spondylosis deformans
- impression of vertebral endplates, crush fractures
- radio-opaque material (iodine, barium)
- metallic dress fastener, calcium tablets
- emission of radiation after recent bone scan

34 What is the relative importance of ultrasound measurement at the calcaneus in comparison to the other methods of densitometry?

Short answer: Sonography of the calcaneus is an interesting screening approach. Most experts, however, do not recommend therapeutic decisions for the individual patient based only on ultrasound results.

Detailed answer: Measurement of the speed of sound and broad band ultrasound attenuation in bone tissue are the basis of quantitative ultrasound (QUS) techniques. Both parameters are supposed to correlate to a certain extent with mechanical strength of bone. In general, the parameter "bone stiffness" is derived from both measurements and is used for the estimation of fracture risk.

There are only moderate correlations between stiffness measured with QUS and the classical DEXA results at the lumbar spine and hip. On the other hand, significant correlations were shown between QUS of the calcaneus and the future risk of hip fracture.

At present, we recommend the use of all different methods of QUS only for a first screening. An expensive long-term therapy of osteoporosis with possible side effects should not be indicated solely on the basis of QUS results.

Further information: QUS methods using other measuring sites (e.g. phalanges, tibia, patella) are less validated than the calcaneus site. Absolutely obsolete is the measurement of skin thickness by ultrasound as a surrogate for bone densitometry (see Question 26).

35 What is the diagnostic value of quantitative CT or DEXA for the staging of osteoporosis?

Short answer: DEXA measurement is today the gold standard of bone densitometry. The WHO fracture thresholds used worldwide were defined for this method, i.e. the best staging can be reached with this method.

Detailed answer: DEXA implies a combined trabecular and cortical bone measurement. Usual measuring sites are the lumbar spine, proximal femur, and total body. The planimetric value in g/cm^2 is strongly correlated to fracture risk. The T score fracture thresholds proposed by the WHO (see Question 20) were made primarily for DEXA. Accordingly, this method is used today in all large international studies as one important parameter for the evaluation of antiosteoporotic drugs.

With quantitative computer tomography (QCT) a volumetric measurement is performed. A separate evaluation of spongy and cortical bone is possible, but mostly the trabecular bone data are used for diagnosis. From our experience the degree of osteoporosis is often overestimated with axial QCT and even more with peripheral QCT at the distal radius when only looking at spongy bone results.

Reproducibility of results is a problem with aQCT and pQCT. If repeated measurements are not done at exactly the same bone section, very discrepant results may be obtained.

36 Is there a chance to improve the identification of high-risk patients by combining BMD results and risk factor assessment?

Short answer: Since fractures always have a multifactorial background the selection of high-risk patients for therapy may be considerably improved by using an algorithm based on BMD and other independent risk factors for fracture.

Detailed answer: Figure **4** shows the multiple factors involved in the fracture risk in the individual patient. The contribution of BMD to fracture risk may differ considerably in different situations. The impact of BMD may be more important in vertebral fractures and lower in hip fracture events.

A working group of the International Osteoporosis Foundation (IOF) is currently collecting suggestions for a combined risk factor/BMD risk score. Independent risk factors could include, e.g. age, low body mass index, previous fractures, maternal fractures (see Question 24).

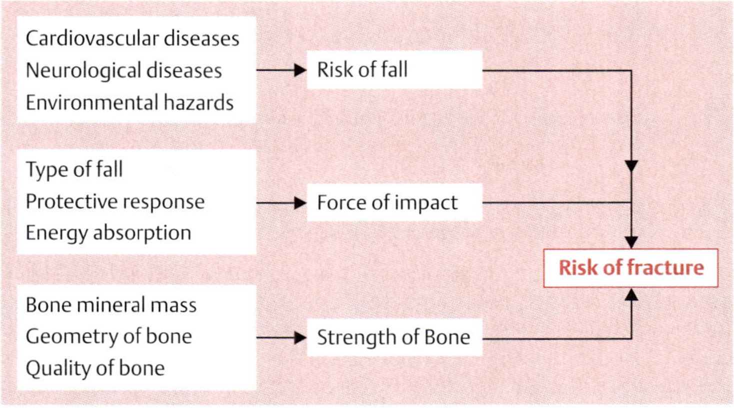

Fig. **4** Multifactorial pathogenesis of fracture risk.

Prevention

37 Can we avoid the development of osteoporosis by a daily program of physical therapy and sports?

Short answer: Regular physical activity or sports with resistance training is able to maintain or increase bone substance.

Detailed answer: The mechanisms of the perception of muscle strain by bone tissue are still not completely understood. It has been proven, however, that bone formation can be increased by augmenting mechanical forces on bone. There have been only few trials which studied the effect of different types of training or sports on BMD so far. There is a general agreement that every kind of resistance training is more effective than limbering-up exercises.

Resistance training programs aiming at stimulation of osteoblastic bone formation should be adapted to age and sex. Optimal levels of physical strain have not been established so far.

Some general advice is given in Table **11** for patients with osteoporosis interested in the potential effects of exercise (see Questions 8 and 9).

Table **11** Physical activity and osteoporosis

- Inactivity favors bone loss and osteoporosis
- Every kind of activity is better than nothing
- Moderate resistance training is suitable to stimulate osteoblastic bone formation
- Every training program should be executed regularly on a daily basis
- Achieved gain of bone substance diminishes very rapidly after stopping a regular training program
- It is never too late: increased mobility has positive effects on muscle and bone also in advanced age
- Gymnastics for the elderly may also reduce fracture risk by reducing the propensity to fall

38 Prevention of osteoporosis: suitable for every patient or based on individual criteria?

Short answer: General measures for the prevention of osteoporosis may be suitable from early childhood until advanced age. Recommendations for every individual case should be made according to risk factors and BMD.

Detailed answer: Avoidance of modifiable individual risk factors is an important first step for the prevention of osteoporosis. With correct information, this can be done by everybody and should be continued for life, e.g. calcium-rich diet, physical activity, avoidance of too much alcohol, tobacco, caffeine.

The three most frequent situations with a specific need for early prevention are postmenopausal, corticoid-induced, and senile osteoporosis:

1. Hormone replacement therapy (HRT) can be recommended to every postmenopausal woman to reduce increased bone turnover. This therapy simultaneously has beneficial effects on climacteric complaints and possibly on the cardiovascular system and the brain. Since a slightly increased risk of breast cancer after a use of HRT for > 5 years cannot be excluded, long-term HRT should not be given to every postmenopausal women but rather to selected cases with clear indications (low BMD, climacteric syndrome, cardiovascular risk factors). Experience shows that the compliance is much better in women with densitometrically proven osteopenia.
2. Patients starting long-term corticosteroid medication should initiate prevention of osteoporosis from the very beginning. The intensity of preventive measures, i.e. the concept of the preventive strategy, depends on the initial BMD, the dosage of corticocoids, and the underlying disease.
3. Calcium and vitamin D deficiencies are extremely frequent in advanced age. A combined calcium/vitamin D supplementation is able to reduce the risk of non-vertebral fractures in the elderly. In patients with mild to moderate impairment of renal function, the activation of cholecalciferol may be delayed. In these patients 0.5 to 1.0 µg of the active D-hormone analogue alfacalcidol should be given instead of 1000 I.U. of plain vitamin D. Recent studies show additional effects of active vitamin D on muscle function, which may further reduce the risk of falls and fracturing.

39 Should estrogen replacement always be combined with progesterone ?

Short answer: The combined cyclic hormone replacement therapy (HRT) with estrogen plus a cyclically administered progestin reduces the risk of endometrial cancer. In hysterectomized women unopposed hormone substitution with estrogen is allowed.

Detailed answer: Continuous treatment with estrogen alone induces permanent stimulation and hyperplasia of the endometrium and may result in malignant transformation. The cyclic combination with a progestin, however, induces regular bleeding, i.e. an initiation of the physiological cycle and a significant reduction of cancer risk. Accordingly, unopposed estrogen is not a problem in women after hysterectomy. Concerning the breast cancer risk, however, neither cyclic nor continuous therapy with estrogen plus progesterone has a proven risk-reducing potency.

Additional information: Among women without HRT, obese subjects have an augmented risk of endometrial cancer development due to higher postmenopausal estrogen levels compared to slim, age-matched controls. The explanation is that the conversion of adrenal androgens by aromatases to estrogen mainly takes place in adipose tissue.

40 What are exclusion criteria or contraindications for HRT ?

Short answer: HRT should not be prescribed in women with breast cancer or thromboembolic disease within the last 5 years.

Detailed answer: There are only few strong contraindications for HRT in postmenopausal women. No estrogen or estrogen/progestin combinations should be given to women having had breast cancer less than 5 years ago and with deep vein thrombosis or pulmonary embolism in their recent history. Endometriosis and endometrial carcinoma are estrogen-dependent diseases and, accordingly, contraindications for HRT.

On the other hand, hypertension and hypercholesterinemia are not contraindications, also often wrongly mentioned in this context. HRT has instead moderate beneficial effects on both conditions.

Women from families with a frequent incidence of breast cancer should not receive HRT.

41 Should hormone replacement therapy (HRT) be adopted in women aged 70 or more years?

Short answer: Estrogens have an inhibitory effect on osteoclastic bone resorption independent of age. An HRT therapy initiated many years previously and well accepted may therefore be continued through to advanced age. Initiation of HRT after the age of 70 years, however, will be rarely accepted.

Detailed answer: The first choice for the prevention of postmenopausal osteoporosis is HRT with estrogen/progesterone or estrogen alone in hysterectomized women. If HRT is stopped after a few years of administration the fracture risk-reducing advantage will terminate 5 years later. HRT has to be taken for at least 8 – 10 years to achieve a long-term benefit for the skeleton.

On the other hand there are epidemiological data reporting a slight increase in breast cancer risk after 5 years of use. Taking these problems into account, a later start at the age of about 70 years could be advocated to reduce the breast cancer risk and to profit from the anti-fracture effects in older age.

In practice, however, a rather large number of women will use HRT early on after menopause for climacteric complaints and then stop after some years. Elderly women rarely accept the re-occurrence of monthly bleeding. The latter problem can be overcome by continuous combined treatment with estrogen and a progestin.

The osteoprotective effect of estrogens persists until very old age and only moderately decreases with aging.

In patients with contraindications for HRT (e.g. families with a high incidence of breast cancer), a selective estrogen receptor modulator (SERM) can be used for prevention or treatment of osteoporosis (raloxifen, 60 mg/day). Another alternative for this indication is a D-hormone analogue (alfacalcidol 1 µg/day).

42 What diagnostic information is needed before starting prevention with antiosteoporotic drugs?

Short answer: The diagnostic prerequisite before starting prevention with specific drugs is the proof of an increased fracture risk.

Detailed answer: Unspecific prevention measures such as changing personal risk factors (nutrition, mobility) can be started without previous diagnostic steps.

Some basic diagnostic information, however, is necessary for prevention using drugs such as calcium/vitamin D and sex steroids or with other specific antiosteoporotic substances such as calcitonin, alfacalcidol, or bisphosphonates.

1. **Diagnostic assessment before calcium/vitamin D supplementation**
   - history of risk factors (prevalent fractures, osteoporosis in family members?)
   - nutrition (dairy products, protein, vegetarian food, sun exposure?)
   - kidney stones (determination of urinary calcium excretion)
   - previous BMD measurements? (not obligatory)
2. **Diagnostic assessment before prevention with sex steroids and other drugs**
   - extensive history of risk factors, history of fractures
   - evaluation of recent BMD measurements
   - laboratory screening (ESR, blood count, Ca, P, alkaline phosphatase, γ-GT, creatinine, electrophoresis
   - marker of bone turnover (e.g. osteocalcin, deoxypyrodinoline)

43 Who are candidates for an antiresorptive therapy with raloxifen?

Short answer: Raloxifen is the first so-called *s*elective *e*strogen *r*eceptor *m*odulator (SERM) approved worldwide for the prevention and treatment of postmenopausal osteoporosis.

Detailed answer: SERMs are a new group of drugs having estrogen-like molecules with differential effects on different target tissues. Raloxifen has effects similar to estrogen on bone tissue and the cardiovascular system but antiestrogenic-antiproliferative effects on breast tissue and endometrium. There is no reduction of climacteric symptoms with raloxifen – rather a slight augmentation (Table **12**).

Based on the excellent results of the large international multicenter MORE study (7705 patients) showing a significant reduction in the in-

Table **12** Characteristics of raloxifen

- approved for prevention and treatment of postmenopausal osteoporosis
- interesting alternative in patients with contraindications for HRT
- can be recommended for women with previous breast cancer or history of breast cancer in the family
- should not be given to women with severe climacteric syndrome
- so far no sufficient clinical experience with male patients
- combination of the antiresorptive raloxifen with anabolic fluoride or PTH will be assessed in an ongoing trials

cidence of vertebral fractures, raloxifen is approved for the prevention and therapy of postmenopausal osteoporosis.

As a result of this study raloxifen has achieved the rating of evidence-based medicine (EBM).

44 State of the art in the prevention of osteoporosis ?

Short answer: There is a general agreement about preventive concepts adapted to the different forms of osteoporosis in different phases of life.

Detailed answer: Avoidance of personal risk factors is a lifelong task. Besides, there are clear recommendations for specific strategies of prevention depending on the age of the patient and the type of osteoporosis.

1. *During childhood:* Balanced diet with high share of calcium-rich dairy products, regular physical activity.
2. *Women in early menopause:* Hormone replacement with estrogen plus cyclic progesterone or estrogen alone in hysterectomized women. Raloxifen in females with increased risk of breast cancer.
3. *Women in later postmenopausal years:* In women aged 60 years and over, without significant risk factors for fracture and mild osteopenia, calcium/vitamin D supplementation may often be sufficient for prevention,
4. *Men aged 40 to 65 years with moderately increased risk and no hypogonadism:* Well balanced calcium-rich alimentation, increase of physical activity, reduction of nicotine and alcohol.

5. *Women and men in advanced age:* Calcium/vitamin D supplementation to reduce the risk of hip fractures; information and practical recommendations to avoid risk factors for falls; in high risk patients hip protector.

Treatment

Basic Treatment, Analgesic Therapy

45 What does the term "basic treatment" of osteoporosis mean?

Short answer: With the term "basic treatment", the simple, first-step measures of the therapeutic concept are summarized. They should be initiated in every patient with osteoporosis, independent of type and clinical stage and imply counteracting changeable risk factors.

Detailed answer: It is not sufficient to prescribe just one potent drug to counteract osteoporosis. The physician in charge should always try to design an adequate, individually adapted therapeutic strategy. In each patient with densitometric, radiological, and clinical proof of osteoporosis, a thorough history of risk factors must be done (see Question 42). Risk factors that are changeable (Table **13**) should be stopped or at least be reduced to the lowest possible level. Based on the detailed anamnesis, recommendations for individual basic treatment should be given within an extended informative discussion with the patient. Of special importance is information about nutrition and exercise.

In most patients it will become evident after a few specific questions that there is a deficit in calcium and vitamin D supplies, which will be difficult to correct just by changes in behavior. In the majority of patients a calcium/vitamin supplementation must be prescribed within the basic treatment.

Table **13** Changeable risk factors

- inactivity, reduced mobility
- low calcium diet (rare intake of dairy products)
- vitamin D insufficiency (rarely fish and/or sunshine)
- nicotine, caffeine, alcohol
- estrogen deficiency (amenorrhea, early menopause)
- long-term corticoid or heparin therapy

46 Are kidney stones a contraindication for calcium/vitamin D supplementation?

Short answer: In patients with a history of kidney stones the renal calcium excretion should be measured in order to adapt the calcium supplementation. A low-calcium diet may increase the risk of calcium-oxalate concrements.

Detailed answer: The risk of kidney stones is not increased with the usual doses of calcium and vitamin D given as a basic treatment of osteoporosis (e.g. 1200 mg calcium, 800 IU vitamin D). An exception is idiopathic hypercalcuria which is observed very rarely in women and somewhat more frequently in men. Urinary calcium can be determined from 24-hour urine or in the morning spot urine and should be related to creatinine excretion. A general screening for hypercalcuria before calcium or calcium/vitamin D supplementation is not necessary.

We recommend, however, measurement of urinary calcium in patients with actual kidney stones or a history of nephrolithiasis to decide whether the calcium and/or vitamin D supplementation should be reduced or omitted.

It has to be stressed that an omission of supplements may be indicated but not the recommendation of a low calcium diet. The latter will lead to calcium deficiency, secondary hyperparathyroidism, and increased bone resorption without reducing the risk of kidney stones. The development of oxalate-containing concrements, the most common type of nephrolithiasis, will even be favored since the resorption of oxalate is increased with a low calcium diet.

47 Analgesic drug therapy of pain after acute new vertebral fractures or progressive fractures?

Short answer: A combined treatment regimen with peripherally and centrally acting analgesic drugs possibly additionally combined with muscle-relaxant substances and calcitonin to avoid immobility depending on the pain is recommended.

Detailed answer: Peripherally acting analgesics (e.g. paracetamol, novaminsulfone, NSAID) are often not sufficient for the acute severe pain after fresh vertebral fractures or "progressive sintering" of vertebrae. We frequently observed a rather good pain reduction by an alternate treatment with novaminsulfone and tramadolol every 4–6 hours. In cases of more severe pain a continuous percutaneous treatment by a fentanyl patch is very effective if the possible adverse events are tolerable. In the individual case the analgesic treatment can be done with different combinations of peripherally or centrally acting drugs according to the respective efficacy, tolerance, and adverse reactions. A combination with muscle relaxants, antidepressive drugs, or calcitonin may help to reduce the dosages of the specific analgesic drugs.

It is of great importance to avoid a partial or total immobilization of the patient as a consequence of the severe pain syndrome. The vicious circle of pain, immobility, and progressive osteoporosis (Fig. **5**) must be interrupted.

During treatment with NSAID, a protective therapy for the stomach (e.g. omeprazole) is mandatory, especially in patients with a history of gastritis or ulcer.

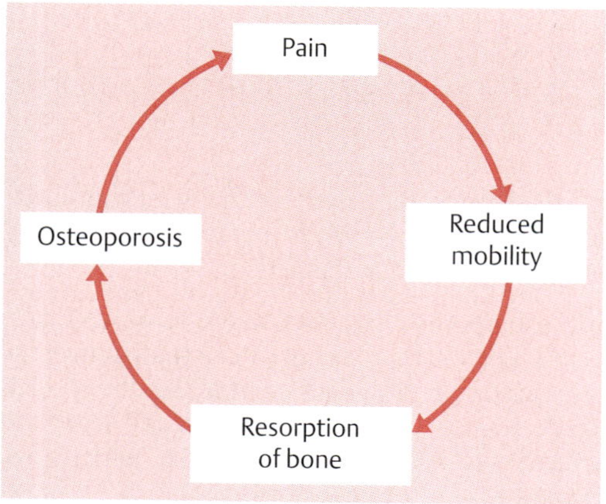

Fig. **5** The vicious circle of pain, immobility and progressive osteoporosis.

48 What is the mechanism of the rapid pain reduction after calcitonin administration?

Short answer: Independent of specific antiosteoclastic effects, calcitonin has an analgesic potency by acting on specific central nervous receptors and, possibly, additional peripheral mechanisms.

Detailed answer: A pain-reducing effect after intracerebroventricular injection of calcitonin was shown for the first time in 1961 in a trial on conscious rabbits by Pecile in Milano. Numerous subsequent publications described more or less impressive analgesic effects in different skeletal and non-skeletal pain syndromes. Later studies pointed out that this was not only true for injection or infusion of the hormone but also for the nasal spray. Large placebo-controlled studies, however, have not been performed to date.

The colleague who posed this question has obviously had very positive experiences with calcitonin in this context. From our own clinical experience and the literature it must be summarized that the pain reduction in, e.g. patients with osteoporosis, algodystrophy, or Paget's disease will occur only after some days even up to two weeks. In cases with a positive response, a reduction of the pain medication can be started step by step.

The respective rates of responders and non-responders to calcitonin with different indications are discussed very controversially in the literature (see analgesic effect of bisphosphonates, Questions 69/70).

49 Pain management of osteoporosis: beneficial effects of bed rest and fitting with a corset?

Short answer: Even after a fresh vertebral fracture with severe pain, long-term bed rest should be avoided. A short-term fitting with a corset may be helpful to facilitate early mobilization of the patient.

Detailed answer: In pure osteoporotic fractures there is no risk of a transverse lesion of the cord (in contrast to traumatic or malignancy induced vertebral fractures with frequent involvement of the dorsal edge of the vertebrae). The classic surgical principle of bed rest and complete immobilization for 4 to 6 weeks is not necessary in patients with osteoporosis and is even detrimental.

In numerous case reports, it has clearly been shown that bone loss increases dramatically during bed rest and that with remobilization after several weeks there is a highly increased risk of further fractures.

After a fresh vertebral fracture, the patient should receive an adequate, individually adapted analgesic treatment (see Question 47) and should leave the bed within a few days.

In principle, the same is true for the use of the different types of corsets. A stabilization and support may be helpful to control pain and speed up mobilization. With long-term use, however, a progressive atrophy of the trunk muscles will occur followed by a corresponding loss of bone substance.

The very rigid, three-point ortheses are rarely tolerated by the patients due to pain at the contact points. If we use any corset at all, we prefer short-term fitting with an elastic corset, correcting mainly the "balloon function" of the abdomen.

50 Under what circumstances must opiates be given in patients with osteoporosis?

Short answer: The management of severe, unbearable back pain immediately after vertebral fractures is often only possible by using opiates.

Detailed answer: Patients report acute, severe back pain after fresh vertebral fractures as mostly unbearable. A large number of our patients suffering simultaneously from coronary heart disease have described the fracture pain as less tolerable than the pain of myocardial infarction. Accordingly, bed rest can mostly not be avoided during the first days.

Since immobility will induce further bone loss, a consequent pain reducing therapeutic regimen must be initiated. In general, we start with a combination of peripherally acting analgesics (paracetamol, novaminsulfone) and NSAID (diclofenac, rofecoxib) but very soon have to proceed to opiates in most patients.

The aim of the therapeutic strategy (which may include physiotherapy and sometimes corset supply) is to reach a rapid pain relief, to start mobilization of the patient, and to avoid further bone loss (see Question 47: vicious circle of pain and osteoporosis).

51 Therapeutic management of osteoporosis: what are today's therapeutic options and how should they be used?

Short answer: Basic treatment, analgesic therapy, antiresorptive and/or osteoanabolic drugs can be used, individually adapted to type and severity of osteoporosis.

Detailed answer: Figure **6** gives a schematic overview of the therapeutic options for patients with osteoporosis. An analgesic therapy has to be added in patients with established disease and back pain (see Questions 47 and 49).

The therapeutic strategy for the individual patient must be planned considering age, sex, pain, fractures, type of osteoporosis, concomitant

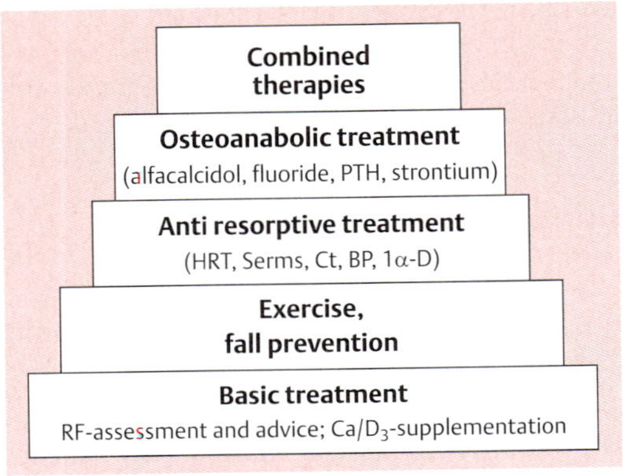

Fig. **6** Therapeutic options for osteoporosis.

diseases and medications, previous treatment, previous adverse events, and expected compliance.

1. Basic treatment comprises risk factor analysis and corresponding recommendations. The most important information to be obtained relates to a sufficient calcium/vitamin D supply.
2. Regular exercise is of high importance to maintain bone mass. In elderly patients possible risk factors for falling should be discussed.
3. Antiresorptive drugs are the first choice in patients with proven high turnover or after recent vertebral fractures with a high risk of subsequent fractures. For alfacalcidol, simultaneous antiresorptive and anabolic effects have been documented.
4. Fluoride, a potent bone formation stimulating agent, is only available in a few countries. We expect that parathyroid hormone and strontium will be introduced as new bone anabolic substances in the near future. Further candidates may be growth hormone and statins. For the latter, significant anabolic and antiresorptive effects were shown in animal studies.
5. Very promising are combinations of anabolic and antiresorptive drugs but large studies are lacking. Positive effects on BMD were documented for fluoride and HRT as well as for alfacalcidol and HRT. Results from first small trials with bisphosphonates plus fluoride are very encouraging.

52 Is calcitonin a valuable treatment?

Short answer: The natural peptide hormone calcitonin inhibits osteoclastic bone resorption. Additional analgesic effects have been described for both subcutaneous and nasal administration.

Detailed answer: Calcitonin is a peptide hormone composed of 32 amino acids, which binds to specific surface receptors of the osteoclast. The resulting antiresorptive effect induces a mild short-term lowering of serum calcium and a long-term moderate increase in BMD.

The antiresorptive potency is less expressed than those of bisphosphonates. On the other hand, salmon and human calcitonin are physiological hormones which are rapidly degraded and will not be deposited in the skeleton. Accordingly, no toxic side effects have been described for calcitonins. They may even be administered without risk to children and in pregnant women.

Until recently, a fracture-reducing efficacy had not been proven for long-term calcitonin therapy. Results of the very recently published 5-year PROOF study on 1255 patients show a significant reduction of vertebral fractures of 36% when using a dosage of 200 IU calcitonin as a nasal spray.

The analgesic potency of calcitonin was described in numerous studies for different types of pain, but was discussed controversially in some reviews (see Question 48). Those who have observed impressive analgesic effects are convinced while others remain skeptical.

All in all, calcitonin can still be considered as an interesting therapeutic option in the increasing choice of drugs against osteoporosis.

Fluorides

53 What is the reason for the discrepant results from different fluoride trials? Is there a consensus about fluoride treatment?

Short answer: Relatively small studies with different fluoride salts and dosages have resulted in contradictory results in the past.

Detailed answer: The first larger fluoride study with a fracture rate as a primary end point was performed in the Mayo Clinic on 135 women with established postmenopausal osteoporosis and published in 1990. A highly significant increase of BMD was observed at the lumbar spine of 36% after 4 years of therapy but no significant effect was seen on the vertebral fracture rate.

Today, it is generally accepted that the 35 mg of bioavailable fluoride per day used in that specific study was much too high. From some patients, bone specimens became available after publication and determinations of the fluoride content in bone tissue showed toxic concentrations comparable to fluorosis (personal communication, Prof. P. J. Meunier, Lyon).

Since then, at least six acceptable, medium-size studies have been performed in Europe and USA using doses between 12 – 25 mg fluoride per day. All but one showed a significant reduction of vertebral fractures.

We assume that doses of 15 – 20 mg of bioavailable fluoride (given as sodium fluoride or monofluorophosphate) may represent the optimal therapeutic range. Combining fluoride with calcium/vitamin D or, even more, with the active analogue alfacalcidol helps to avoid undermineralization of newly formed bone substance, i.e. makes fluoride a safer treatment [1].

There is as yet no international consensus about the therapeutic value of fluoride treatment. Large studies with more than 1000 patients are still lacking and probably will never be undertaken. The problem of fluoride is the very low price and the lack of patent protection, i.e. there is no interest in performing such an expensive trial. Fluoride is an orphan drug.

Reference

1 Ringe JD. Fluoride in osteoporosis. In: Principles of Bone Biology (second edition). Eds.: JP Bilezikian, LG Raisz, GA Rodan. Academic Press, San Diego, 2001

54 Adverse events during fluoride therapy?

Short answer: During long-term fluoride treatment, gastrointestinal irritations and a lower limb pain syndrome may occur. These drug-related adverse events are rare with the doses and galenic preparations used today.

Detailed answer:

1. *Gastrointestinal side effects:* When using plain sodium fluoride (NaF) there is a rather high risk of epigastric complaints. The salt dissociates in the presence of HCl in the stomach and free fluoride ions irritate the mucosa. With retarded/enterocoated NaF these side effects are rare and moderate. Using monofluorophosphate (MFP) gastrointestinal side effects are very infrequent since fluoride is resorbed in the form of an entire fluorophosphates ion in the proximal gut.
2. *Lower extremity pain syndrome:* During fluoride treatment, patients sometimes complain about acute pain mainly in the region of the ankle, rarely at the knee or the hip region. Histological studies revealed undermineralized microcallus formation as the correlate of this so-called lower extremity pain syndrome (LEPS). After interruption of therapy, pain will diminish within 4 – 6 weeks.
3. *Iatrogenic fluorosis:* This is not an adverse drug reaction but results always from treatment mistakes. Fluoride is given at too high a dose for too long a time or to patients with an unfounded suspicion of osteoporosis, i.e. normal BMD (see Question 55).

55 Long-term fluoride treatment: How can iatrogenic fluorosis be avoided?

Short answer: The development of fluorosis can be avoided by adequate dosage, regular controls of BMD, and a timely limitation of treatment.

Detailed answer: Endemic fluorosis is a disease characterized by a generalized pathological hyperostosis or osteosclerosis due to lifelong consumption of drinking water with a very high fluoride content. In severe cases, calcification of tendons and ligaments can be observed.

Iatrogenic fluorosis is always the result of an erroneous therapy. Uncontrolled long-term use of rather high doses of fluoride may result in an overstimulation of osteoblasts and pathologically increased bone density. In some patients we have found a lumbar spine BMD of 200% and more compared to age-matched controls. In these cases the diagnosis can be made from X-rays showing "white vertebrae".

A very important role is obviously played by the prevalent bone mass at the onset of fluoride medication. In patients with the erroneous diagnosis of osteoporosis (based, for example, on X-rays of poor quality), but indeed having a normal BMD, fluorosis may develop very rapidly. It is suggested that the large endosteal surface allows an excessive formation of new bone in these patients.

There is no evidence whether an individual predisposition increases the risk of fluorosis but there are some data suggesting that the simultaneous ingestion of aluminium-containing drugs can accelerate fluorosis.

Follow-up after cessation of fluoride therapy shows a slow diminishing of hyperostosis over several years. We have never observed pathological fractures in patients with iatrogenic fluorosis.

Table **14** Avoidance of iatrogenic fluorosis

- Correct clinical, densitometric, and radiological diagnosis of osteoporosis
- Dosage of NaF or MFP corresponding to 15–20 mg of bioavailable fluoride ions per day.
- Limitation of treatment duration to 3–4 years.
- Control of BMD and blood chemistry every year (increase of alkaline phosphatase?)
- X-ray controls are insufficient (first visibility on X-ray corresponds already to stage I fluorosis).

56 Are there data supporting the combined use of fluoride with bisphosphonates? Higher increase in BMD, better bone quality?

Short answer: The combination of anabolic fluoride and antiresorptive bisphosphonates is an interesting therapeutic approach, especially in advanced cases of osteoporosis. However, it is not evidence-based medicine.

Detailed answer: The increase of BMD during treatment with antiresorptive drugs is limited and a plateau may be reached during the third or fourth year when using bisphosphonates. The increase in BMD mainly reflects a higher degree of mineralization but not a true gain in bone mass.

It is an important and not definitely answered question whether the well documented continuous increase of bone mass during controlled fluoride therapy may be optimized by cyclic intermittent or continuous parallel combination with bisphosphonates.

First small trials with etidronate plus NaF in corticoid-induced and postmenopausal osteoporosis showed significantly higher increases of BMD than with each drug given alone.

In two pilot studies in postmenopausal women and in men with severe established osteoporosis we used etidronate 400 mg/day for 14 days followed by 76 days with 20 mg fluoride (from MFP) plus a calcium/vitamin D supplement and confirmed additive effects on lumbar spine and hip BMD.

Additional information: More recent studies with continuous combined fluoride/alendronate show similar effects on BMD. For definite evaluation of the therapeutic value of these treatments fracture data and histological studies are required.

Alfacalcidol

57 What are the differences and advantages of alfacalcidol versus plain vitamin D ?

Short answer: Plain vitamin D will only show effects on calcium metabolism and bone mineral density in patients with preexisting vitamin D deficiency.

Alfacalcidol is hydroxylated in the liver to 1,25-dihydroxycholecalciferol, the highly active D-hormone, with specific effects on the gut, bone, parathyroid glands, and several other tissues.

Detailed answer: Plain vitamin D in high doses is effective in healing rickets and osteomalacia, i.e. diseases with severe vitamin D deficiency or resistance. In selected populations of elderly people with low vitamin D levels (vitamin D insufficiency) it will decrease PTH, slightly increase BMD, and thereby reduce the risk of fractures.

In the large number of osteoporotic patients who are replete in vitamin D, no significant effects can be expected from plain vitamin D. Nevertheless, very often calcium plus vitamin D supplements are given just to guarantee an optimal supply.

Also in patients under long-term corticoid therapy it has been shown that calcium plus plain vitamin D alone has no significant effect on BMD [1].

After intestinal absorption alfacalcidol will readily be activated in the liver into 1,25-dihydroxycholecalciferol (= calcitriol), i.e. the plasma level of this active hormone will be augmented inducing effects on calcium absorption, PTH, and bone turnover. This will never occur even with rather high doses of plain vitamin D because the second activation step in the kidney (1α-hydroxylase) is strongly regulated. Alfacalcidol, however, is already 1α-hydroxylated, and activation in the liver will take place quantitatively without regulation.

Table **15** summarizes the most important differences between plain vitamin D and the active analogue alfacalcidol.

From a therapeutic point of view plain vitamin D can be used as a nutritional supplement in case of insufficient supply, while alfacalcidol is a specific antiosteoporotic drug.

Table **15** Plain vitamin D or active alfacalcidol?

Plain vitamin D – Nutritional substitution	Alfacalcidol – Pharmacological treatment
– Only effective in patients with vitamin D insufficiency	– Prodrug for calcitriol, will be activated in the liver and in bone
– In vitamin D replete patients no further increase of 1,25-$(OH)_2$-D (calcitriol) takes place	– Resulting increase in active D-hormone will decrease PTH and bone resorption, and increase formation

Reference

1 Ringe JD, Faber H. Calcium and vitamin D in the prevention and treatment of glucocorticoid-induced osteoporosis. Clin Exp Rheumatol 2000; 18 Suppl 21: S44–S48

58 What is the rationale for using alfacalcidol in corticosteroid-induced, senile, post-transplantation, and postmenopausal osteoporosis ?

Short answer: Alfacalcidol increases intestinal calcium absorption, reduces hyperactivity of parathyroid glands, decreases bone resorption, and stimulates osteoblastic bone formation. Accordingly beneficial effects have been reported in all mentioned types of osteoporosis.

Detailed answer: The prodrug alfacalcidol is hydroxylated in the liver to the active D-hormone (see Question 57). The different effects of this very potent hormone are listed in Table **16**.

Several studies from Europe show very positive effects especially in corticoid-induced osteoporosis [1, 2] and in post-organ transplantation osteoporosis. In the latter the immunological effects of alfacalcidol may play an additional role and deserve further investigation.

The high risk of hip fracture in senile osteoporosis can be reduced by alfacalcidol. There is increasing evidence that the positive effects of the D-hormone on muscle metabolism may reduce the risk of falling and thereby contribute to the reduction in hip fracture events.

Most of the positive therapeutic experience with alfacalcidol in postmenopausal osteoporosis has been established in Japan.

Table **16** Rationale for using alfacalcidol in different forms of osteoporosis

1. Increase of intestinal calcium absorption after activation in the liver
2. Decrease of PTH secretion by the parathyroid glands (= down-regulation of secondary hyperparathyroidism)
3. Antiresorptive effect on bone tissue by reducing activity of osteoclasts
4. Stimulatory effect on osteoblasts (osteoblasts have D-hormone receptors; alfacalcidol is activated in part locally in bone tissue)
5. Improvement of mineralization of bone matrix and newly formed bone tissue
6. Positive effects on muscle metabolism and neuromuscular coordination (muscle cells have D-hormone receptors)
7. Immunosuppressive, immunomodulatory, and antiproliferative effects

References

1 Ringe JD, Cöster A, Meng T, Schacht E, Umbach R. Treatment of glucocorticoid-induced osteoporosis with alfacalcidol/calcium versus vitamin D/calcium. Calcif Tissue Int 1999; 63: 337 – 340

2 Reginster JY, Kuntz D, Verdickt W, Wouters M, Guillevi L, Menkes CJ, Nielsen K. Prophylactic use of alfacalcidol in corticosteroid-induced osteoporosis. Osteoporos Int 1999; 9: 75 – 81

59 Are there clinically relevant differences between alfacalcidol and calcitriol ?

Short answer: *Pharmacodynamic difference:* After oral ingestion calcitriol will partly bind directly to specific receptors of the intestinal mucosa and increase calcium absorption. Alfacalcidol is absorbed by intestinal cells and transported by the portal system to the liver. Only after hepatic 25-hydroxylation will it exert its hormonal effects.

Detailed answer: The D-analogue alfacalcidol (1α-hydroxycholecalciferol) is a prodrug of calcitriol (= 1,25-dihydroxycholecalciferol). After intestinal absorption alfacalcidol is readily hydroxylated in the liver to 1,25-dihydroxycholecalciferol, i.e. the active D-hormone (see Question 63, Fig. **8**: special situation of alfacalcidol bypassing the kidney activation step). Interestingly there are data showing that the activation takes place to some extent also in bone tissue. This *in vivo* activation of alfacalcidol in liver and bone has some advantages:

- The increased intestinal calcium absorption is somewhat retarded, i.e. there is a lower risk of transient hypercalcemia and/or hypercalciuria as compared with primary administration of calcitriol.
- The amount of alfacalcidol that is activated in the bone tissue may increase the local osteoblastic activity.

These findings provide an important therapeutic advantage because the pro-drug technique offers greater pharmacological benefit and a wider therapeutic range due to continuous transformation to the active metabolite and constant distribution in a physiological dose to all target organs, and particularly for bone and parathyroid glands.

Table **17** Differences between calcitriol and alfacalcidol

Calcitriol	Alfacalcidol
– After oral intake absorption or immediate binding to small intestinal receptors	– After oral intake absorption and activation mainly in the liver (25-hydroxylation)
– Plasma peaks of calcitriol and increased risk of hypercalcemia and hypercalciuria	– Balanced plasma curve of calcitriol; lower risk of hypercalciuria and hypercalcemia
	– Advantage of additional activation in bone tissue

60 What are the mechanisms for the fracture reducing potency of alfacalcidol?

Short answer: Although large studies are still lacking there is accumulated evidence today that long-term treatment with alfacalcidol is able to significantly reduce the rate of new vertebral fractures. The contributing mechanisms are inhibition of bone resorption, stimulation of osteoblasts, and increase in muscle strength.

Detailed answer: Taking together all prospective controlled studies performed with alfacalcidol in postmenopausal and corticoid-induced osteoporosis shows a clear reduction of vertebral fractures. In a separate study on hip fractures there was a significant effect of the D-analogue compared to placebo in reducing this type of fracture.

In contrast to other antiosteoporotic drugs, which have either antiresorptive or anabolic effects, alfacalcidol obviously acts by different additive mechanisms. The main effects at the level of the gut and parathyroid glands, and of bone and muscle resulting finally in a reduced fracture rate are shown in Figure **7**.

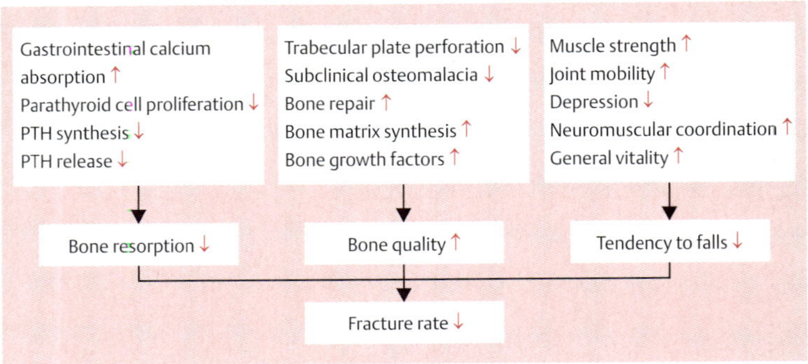

Fig. **7** Mechanisms for the fracture-reducing efficacy of alfacalcidol.

61 Combination of alfacalcidol with other drugs?

Short answer: Different combinations are possible (HRT, raloxifen, calcitonin, fluoride, bisphosphonates), but only small pilot studies have been carried out so far. Preliminary results are encouraging.

Detailed answer: Since alfacalcidol has antiresorptive and anabolic effects, all other anabolic and antiresorptive drugs are potential candidates for combined trials to evaluate whether additive effects can be achieved. Most of the possible combinations have not been studied by prospective controlled trials.

For the combination alfacalcidol/fluoride positive effects on the quality of newly formed bone substance were reported in the literature, but confirming data are still lacking.

The so far largest study has been performed by C. Gallagher with active vitamin D plus HRT. The effect on BMD was significantly higher than with HRT alone.

In a pilot study from our group 12 men with established idiopathic osteoporosis were treated with the combination alendronate/alfacalcidol/calcium at the respective doses of 10 mg/1 µg/500 mg. The increase in BMD at the lumbar spine and femoral neck after 12 months was significantly higher than with alendronate/calcium or alfacalcidol/calcium given separately.

Based on our clinical experience, we recommend combined treatment regimens, especially in very advanced cases of osteoporosis or in "treatment-resistant" patients. Alfacalcidol is a very interesting partner for all kinds of combinations due to its different effects on calcium metabolism, bone and muscle (see Question 58, Table **16**).

62 How safe is alfacalcidol during long-term therapy?

Short answer: No toxic or teratogenic side effects have been reported for the vitamin D analogue alfacalcidol. There is a moderately augmented risk for hypercalciuria and a very low risk for hypercalcemia. These risks may increase with the amount of oral calcium intake.

Detailed answer: Before starting a long-term treatment with alfacalcidol serum and urinary calcium should be controlled and the patient should be interviewed concerning his/her average daily consumption of calcium-rich nutrients (milk, milk products, calcium supplements, plain vitamin D).

Significant hypercalcemia or hypercalciuria and recent kidney stones are, of course, contraindications for alfacalcidol.

If the daily calcium intake is above 1000 mg, no additional calcium should be given. At average intakes between 400–600 mg/day a supplement of 500 mg is recommended. In general, the daily supplement of calcium together with alfacalcidol should not exceed 500 mg.

Controls of urinary calcium should be performed at regular intervals during long-term alfacalcidol treatment.

Altogether, alfacalcidol is a safe drug and the risk of increases in serum or urinary calcium is very small when following the above recommendations.

63 Prevention and treatment of secondary hyperparathyroidism in chronic renal insufficiency?

Short answer: Alfacalcidol plus calcium carbonate is an approved treatment to increase lowered serum calcium, to reduce secondary hyperparathyroidism and the risk of renal bone disease in patients with chronic renal failure.

Detailed answer: The major pathogenetic factors inducing renal bone disease in patients with chronic renal insufficiency before or during hemodialysis are low serum calcium and increased phosphorus leading to secondary hyperparathyroidism .

The aim of prevention or treatment is to normalize both parameters. This can be achieved by alfacalcidol increasing serum calcium. The increasing trends in calcium level and the direct effects of alfacalcidol on the parathyroid glands will reduce PTH secretion. The addition of calcium carbonate will further slightly increase serum calcium and decrease serum phosphorus.

In complex forms of renal osteodystrophy with histological features of hyperparathyroidism and osteomalacia, alfacalcidol not only normalizes the former but also will improve the mineralization of the osteomalacic bone.

Plain vitamin D and 25-hydroxycholecalciferol are not indicated for prevention or therapy of renal bone disease. Both substances will not be sufficiently activated in patients with renal failure or nephrectomy.

Figure **8** shows the metabolism of vitamin D in general and the special situation of alfacalcidol bypassing the activation step in the kidney.

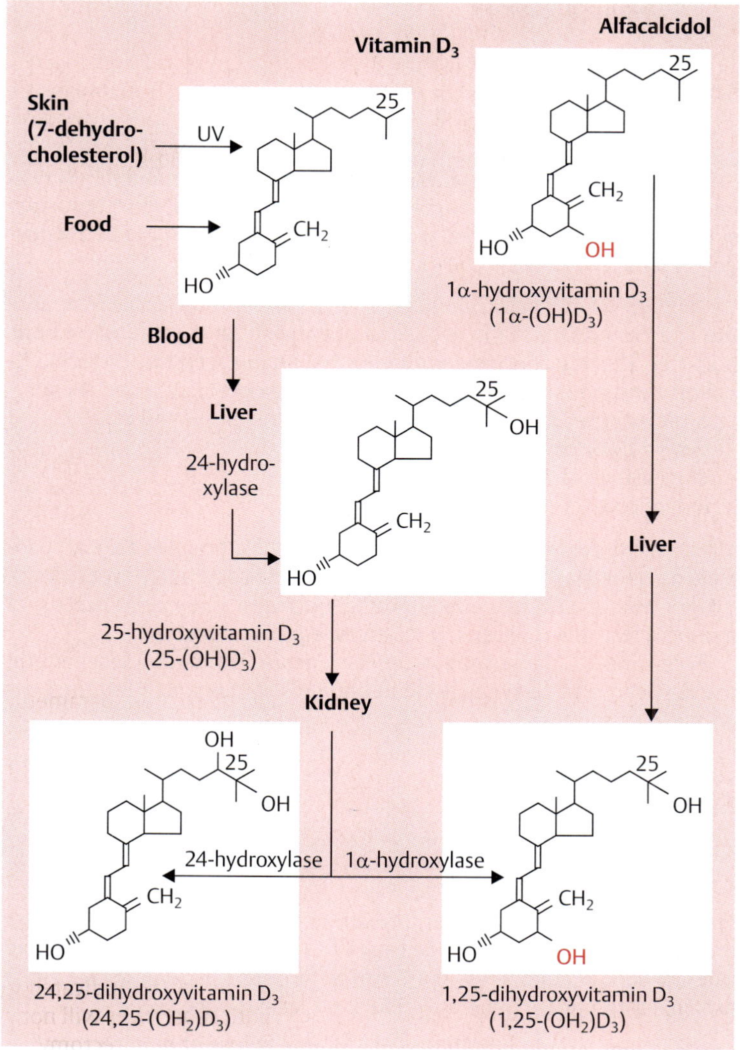

Fig. **8** Metabolism of vitamin D and alfacalcidol.

Bisphosphonates

64 What are the effects of bisphosphonates on bone cells and bone turnover?

Short answer: Bisphosphonates inhibit active osteoclasts and the recruitment of new osteoclasts. As a consequence, a rapid and distinct reduction of bone resorption occurs and with some delay there will also be a reduction in bone formation.

Detailed answer: Bisphosphonates have a high affinity for hydroxyapatite and are preferentially deposited at bone surfaces with active bone turnover. This effect is used for bone scans: main accretion of technetium bisphosphonate in areas with active bone destruction and repair.

After incorporation of bisphosphonates osteoclasts will exhibit:

- vanishing of basal brush border,
- decreasing secretion of acid and proteases,
- loss of contact to bone, apoptosis.

More recent data support the idea that bisphosphonates also have effects on osteoblasts. A decrease in osteoblastic secretion of specific cytokines was described, which would normally induce the fusion of mononuclear macrophages to multinuclear preosteoclasts.

According to these cellular effects, measurement of biochemical markers show an early decrease in bone resorption and a retarded decrease in formation.

65 Bisphosphonate therapy: increase in bone mass or only in bone density and how to explain the significant positive effect on fractures?

Short answer: During long-term treatment with bisphosphonates there is mainly an increase in bone density. The reason for the decreasing fracture incidence could be an amelioration in the microarchitecture and a prolonged secondary mineralization of trabecular bone.

Detailed answer: After inhibition of osteoclastic resorption, recently excavated lacunae will be filled up by osteoblasts, i.e. there is a small initial gain in bone mass. If this occurs at mechanically important areas it may be improve the strength of trabecular bone considerably.

Densitometric controls during bisphosphonate treatment show an increase with a maximum in the first year and a declining increase thereafter. This continuous increase is explained by the permanently reduced bone turnover, i.e. the chance for a prolonged secondary mineralization of bone tissue (= increase in bone density not mass). This hypothesis is based on quantitative microradiographic studies on bone biopsies by the group of P. Meunier [1].

With the recommended dosage regimens of etidronate, alendronate, and risedronate, however, there is no complete stop of bone turnover with the risk of an "over aged hypermineralized" bone. Interestingly, several large studies show a significant reduction of vertebral fractures already after one year. The rate of fracture reduction of the first year (e.g. 60%) does not increase further during the following years.

Reference

1 Boivin GY, Chavssieux PM, Santora AC, Yates J, Meunier PJ. Alendronate increases bone strength by increasing the mean degree of mineralization of bone tissue in osteoporotic women. Bone 2000; 17: 687–694

66 How long should bisphosphonate treatment be continued?

Short answer: New results with risedronate and retrospective results with alendronate show a significant decrease in the incidence of vertebral fractures after as little as one year. The decision about the duration of active therapy must be made on an individual basis.

Detailed answer: The therapeutic aim in patients with osteoporosis is not to achieve a maximum increase in BMD but to stabilize bone substance and to avoid future fractures and pain. According to the solid clinical experience accumulated in the large international bisphosphonate trials, a three-year treatment can be recommended in severe established osteoporosis. In selected cases, this treatment may be extended for a further 1 to 2 years of therapy. After stopping bisphosphonates, we prescribe a "maintenance treatment" with calcium and vitamin D.

In some cases with moderate osteoporosis a 12-month course of bisphosphonate may be sufficient. Annual BMD controls will indicate whether a new active intervention will become necessary in the following years.

67 Why were bisphosphonates approved only for postmenopausal osteoporosis?

Short answer: On the basis of the patients included in the large international studies etidronate, alendronate and risedronate were approved primarily only for postmenopausal women. With the emerging data on corticoid and male osteoporosis the respective approvals are now in progress.

Detailed answer: Today's policy of health authorities is to approve the use of drugs against osteoporosis only on the basis of the presented study data. Accordingly, all oral bisphosphonates were primarily approved for the treatment of postmenopausal osteoporosis.

For further labels (e.g. prevention, corticoid-induced and male osteoporosis) the corresponding studies are required. Whether it is really necessary from a scientific point of view to prove again the anti-fracture-efficacy or whether equipotency in terms of biochemical markers and BMD is sufficient, is the subject of controversial debate.

In the meantime, the three mentioned bisphosphonates are also approved for corticoid-induced osteoporosis in most countries.

Alendronate was studied in two independent studies on male osteoporosis and was recently approved by the FDA (Food and Drug Administration, USA). As usual other countries will follow very soon.

68 What are the reasons for the considerable differences in antiresorptive potency and adverse events of different bisphosphonates?

Short answer: Differences in length and chemical structure of the larger lateral chain of bisphosphonates are responsible for their respective biological activity and potential adverse events.

Detailed answer: There is a close structural resemblance between synthetic bisphosphonates and natural pyrophosphate: bisphosphonates are analogues of pyrophosphate, containing a carbon instead of an oxygen atom. The P-C-P structure allows a great number of variations by changing the two lateral chains on the carbon atom. Bisphosphonates are resistant to chemical and enzymatic hydrolysis. They have a strong affinity for metal ions, including calcium (Fig. **9**).

A large number of bisphosphonates has been investigated. Each has its own characteristic profile of activity.

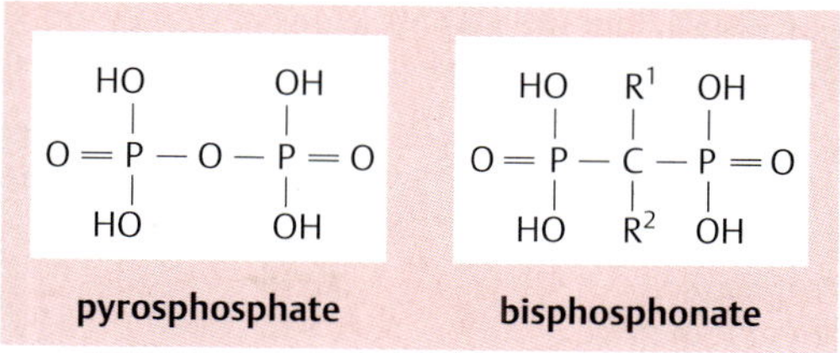

Fig. 9 Structure of pyrophosphate and bisphosphonate.

With increasing length of the lateral chain R^2 the antiresorptive potency increases but simultaneously the intestinal absorption rate declines. The average intestinal absorption rate for etidronate is 2–3%, for alendronate and risedronate below 1%.

Nitrogen or amino groups in the R^2 chain increase the biological activity (e.g. pamidronate, alendronate, risedronate, ibandronate) but also induce a higher rate of gastrointestinal side effects.

Oral administration of these amino-bisphosphonates can be accompanied by esophageal and gastrointestinal symptoms, such as nausea, dyspepsia, vomiting, gastric pain, and diarrhea, and sometimes esophageal erosions or ulcerations. This effect is explained today by the inhibitory effects of nitrogen-containing bisphosphonates on the mevanolate pathway, which leads to an inhibition of keratinocyte growth, or to some direct chemical irritation of mucosa.

69 Treatment of osteoporosis by intravenous bisphosphonates?

Short answer: Up to now we have no intravenous bisphosphonate approved for the treatment of osteoporosis. The intravenous administration is, however, a very attractive concept and the published studies show highly significant effects.

Detailed answer: The therapeutic effect of bisphosphonates depends on the activity of the adopted compound and on the amount deposited on the bone surfaces. The loading of bone tissue can be achieved by small daily oral doses or by intermittent intravenous bolus injections or infusions.

Pamidronate and ibandronate are both approved in many countries for the intravenous treatment of malignant bone disease, but are widely used off label for osteoporosis with the following dosages:

- pamidronate: 30 mg *i.v.* every 3 months by infusion,
- ibandronate: 2 mg *i.v.* every 3 months by injection.

There are several very interesting advantages of *i.v.* bisphosphonate treatment:
- 100% bioavailability,
- no problems with compliance,
- no gastrointestinal adverse events.

We have treated a large number of patients with corticoid-induced osteoporosis with the 2 mg ibandronate regimen. In this cohort of patients we observed a high interest and very good acceptance of the *i.v.* application, most of them having already to swallow a large number of drugs. The effect on BMD and pain relief was highly significant [1].

Reference

1 Ringe JD, Cöster A, Dorst A, Umbach R. Treatment of corticoid-induced osteoporosis by 3-monthly intravenous ibandronate injections. J Bone Miner Res 2000; 15 Suppl 1: 1044

70 Analgesic potency of bisphosphonates

Short answer: A rather fast reduction of pain is observed very often when treating different systemic or localized skeletal diseases with bisphosphonates. An intrinsic analgesic effect has not been documented so far.

Detailed answer: With increased osteoclastic bone resorption, there may be a loss of mechanically important trabecular bone structures with a consequent mechanical insufficiency. Stress and strain will then lead to pain due to reversible bending and deformation of bone.

It is supposed that the rapid inhibition of bone resorption by bisphosphonates induces a rather quick stabilization of trabecular bone architecture and decrease in pain perception. During bisphosphonate therapy of different skeletal disorders a significant improvement of pain has already been noticed after a few days up to several weeks.

Up to now no intrinsic analgesic effect, independent on the effect on bone turnover (similar to calcitonin), could be proved for bisphosphonates. According to clinical experience the analgesic effects may occur earlier with intravenous bisphosphonate administration than with oral intake.

Table **18** Skeletal disorders in which a rather rapid amelioration of bone pain was observed during bisphosphonate therapy

- Metastatic bone disease
- Algodystrophy (Sudeck's atrophy)
- Transient circumscribed osteoporosis
- Fibrous dysplasia, Paget's disease
- Generalized osteoporosis
- Primary hyperparathyroidism

71 Does it make sense to combine hormone replacement treatment (HRT) with bisphophonates ?

Short answer: In patients using HRT for established osteoporosis and climacteric symptoms, the antiresorptive effect on bone can be reinforced by bisphosphonates.

Detailed answer: Although estrogen and bisphosphonates both have antiresorptive activities by inhibiting osteoclasts, additive effects were shown in some studies.

In daily practice there are two distinct scenarios:

1. The established osteoporosis of a postmenopausal woman without climacteric symptoms is treated by a strongly acting antiresorptive bisphosphonate. In this case there is not sufficient evidence that addition of a weaker antiresorptive estrogen will produce long-term beneficial effects.
2. A postmenopausal woman with established osteoporosis has accepted HRT and reports beneficial effects on her climacteric symptoms. In this case there is no reason to stop HRT with the intention of giving a stronger antiresorptive bisphosphonate. The combined antiresorptive-antiresorptive medication may even show moderate additive effects on bone turnover and BMD.

This beneficial effect may also be seen with raloxiden/bisphosphonate. But no effects on climacteric symptoms can be expected.

Further Therapeutic Aspects

72 Should calcium/vitamin D be added to every specific antiosteoporotic treatment?

Short answer: In most elderly patients treatment of osteoporosis should be given together with a calcium/vitamin D supplement. It should not be added automatically, however, but only after checking the individual indication or possible contraindications.

Detailed answer: An insufficient supply of calcium and vitamin D can be found in the majority of elderly people. In patients with established osteoporosis the proportion is even higher than in age-matched healthy controls.

There are two main arguments for giving a calcium/vitamin D supplement to these patients:

1. Calcium/vitamin D insufficiency is an important pathogenetic factor in senile osteoporosis.
2. It has been clearly demonstrated that long-term supplementation with both substances reduces the risk of non-vertebral fractures (see Question 45).

If an insufficient calcium/vitamin D supply can be presumed (nutrition, sunlight exposure), and if hypercalcuria, renal insufficiency, and kidney stones are excluded, Ca/D supplements can be added to every therapeutic regimen, e.g. HRT, SERM, calcitonin, bisphosphonates. With fluoride it is even mandatory.

Exception: When treating osteoporosis with the vitamin D analogue alfacalcidol, the calcium supplementation should be restricted to 500 mg per day. Additional plain vitamin D is not necessary. An exception can be complex osteopathies with secondary hyperparathyroidism and osteomalcia due to intestinal Ca/D malabsorption.

73 What is the role of bone densitometry in treatment control?

Short answer: Back pain, bone densitometry, and fracture incidence are the most important parameters of control during long-term treatment of osteoporosis. A significant increase in BMD is a motivation for the patient to remain on the therapy.

Detailed answer: Theoretically one could omit densitometric control when using a proven effective regimen in a patient with optimal compliance. With every treatment, however, there is a percentage of non-responders and compliance over several years without reinforcement is rare.

If there is a significant decrease of BMD after one or two years of therapy this may be due to non-compliance or indicate a true non-responder. If the latter is the case the treatment regimen could be combined with other substances or completely changed.

Further information: Compliance to treatment can also be checked by measuring biochemical markers of bone turnover (see Question 21). During antiresorptive treatment, markers of bone turnover should be reduced already after 6 to 8 weeks. A rather moderate decrease of markers after 3 months often correlates with a rather small increase of BMD after one year.

74 What is the role of raloxifen in the treatment of osteoporosis? Combination with other substances?

Short answer: Raloxifen is able to reduce the rate of new vertebral fractures in postmenopausal women with preclinical or established osteoporosis.

Detailed answer: Raloxifen was the first SERM (selective estrogen receptor modulator) approved almost worldwide for the treatment of postmenopausal osteoporosis. The increase in lumbar spine BMD of 2–3% is lower than with amino-bisphosphonates but the fracture-reducing potency at the spine is the same (about 50%).

It is our clinical experience that acceptance and compliance to raloxifen are very high in well-informed women. It is important to underline that raloxifen is not an estrogen but a new and very interesting compound with a distinct antiosteoporotic potency besides other beneficial effects (e.g. antiatherosclerotic, reduction of breast cancer risk, see Question 43).

As with other drugs, raloxifen should be given together with a calcium supplement or with Ca/D in the elderly.

A combined treatment of raloxifen with other specific substances could further improve the therapeutic results. So far, however, no clinical experience has been published.

Due to the different mechanisms of action we believe that the combination raloxifen/alfacalcidol could be very effective. We have started a corresponding study giving 60 mg raloxifen, 1 µg alfacalcidol, and 500 mg calcium per day to women with established postmenopausal osteoporosis.

75 What is the perspective of patients with severe established osteoporosis? Is there a chance of stopping the disease and improving quality of life?

Short answer: An individually adapted therapeutic strategy including change of lifestyle according to risk factors, analgesic therapy, and long-term specific osteological medication is able to improve the skeletal status and the quality of life.

Detailed answer: Even today osteoporosis is regarded by most patients and often by inexperienced doctors as an untreatable progressive disease. This is a very common error.

The classical situation of established osteoporosis with significantly reduced BMD values, vertebral fractures, chronic back pain, and typical changes in stature can be stopped by a consistent and long-term treatment. Very often we observe just the contrary: insufficient medication with frequent changes of compounds due to fear and insufficient knowledge of therapeutic options and possible adverse events.

It is very important to tailor a therapeutic strategy for every patient adapted to age, sex, stage of disease, contributing risk factors, pain, etc.

This strategy should comprise basic measures (see Question 45), analgesic therapy (see Question 47), and a controlled long-term use of one or more specific antiosteoporotic drugs (see Question 51).

Treatment monitoring at regular intervals will show whether modifications become necessary.

Senile Osteoporosis

76 What has to be taken into consideration when treating osteoporosis in advanced age?

Short answer: The therapeutic concept must be planned very carefully taking into account biological age, stage of osteoporosis, risk of future fractures, complaints, quality of life, comorbidity, and life expectancy.

Detailed answer: In very aged patients with osteoporosis it is important to assess a number of disease-related, multimorbidity-related and socioeconomic aspects before designing a useful and acceptable therapeutic concept for the individual patient.

Some special aspects for management of senile osteoporosis are listed below:

1. Established osteoporosis of the spine with multiple vertebral fractures may be inactive and asymptomatic in the elderly. Lumbar spine BMD can be rather high due to fractures and degenerative changes. Sometimes no specific therapy is necessary.
2. BMD results from the proximal femur are often more relevant than spine measurements. In spite of "normal" BMD at the spine, treatment may be indicated to decrease the risk of hip fracture.
3. Treatment of active painful osteoporosis at the spine should focus on analgesics and physiotherapy. A specific long-term bone turnover modifying therapy requires a strong indication.
4. In patients with advanced multimorbidity, dementia, and reduced life expectancy the initiation of an, e.g. 3-year bisphosphonate regimen may not be indicated.
5. We have seen good therapeutic results in females with severe senile osteoporosis under daily calcium/vitamin D supplements and intramuscular injections of 50 mg nandrolone decanoate every 3 weeks.
6. In patients with frequent falls in the past, a hip protector can reduce the risk of hip fracture by 50%.

77 Are there specific pathogenetic mechanisms in senile osteoporosis which could be pivotal for treatment?

Short answer: Due to an insufficient calcium/vitamin D supply in persons of advanced age there is a high prevalence of secondary hyperparathyroidism which enhances bone resorption and fracture risk.

Detailed answer: Epidemiological studies in many countries have clearly shown that the rate of low 25-OH-D blood levels increases with age and that the percentage of hypovitaminosis D at age 80 years and over may amount to 95% (Table **19**).

In two independent studies it has been shown that calcium/vitamin D supplements given to 70–80-year-old healthy persons increase vitamin D levels, decrease PTH, and reduce the rate of non-vertebral and hip fractures by about 40% [1, 2].

Table **19** Factors contributing to the high prevalence of hypovitaminosis D and calcium deficits in the elderly

1. Reduced consumption of milk and milk products
2. Decreasing absorption capacity of intestinal mucosa with age
3. Very little or no vitamin D supply with alimentation (especially no fat sea fish)
4. Rare or no exposure of skin to sun
5. Reduced efficacy of old skin to synthesize vitamin D compared to young persons

References

1 Chapuy MC, Arlot ME, DuBoef F, Brun J, Crouzet B, Arnaud S, Delmas PD, Meunier PJ. Vitamin D3 and calcium to prevent hip fractures in elderly women. N Engl J Med 1992; 327: 1637–1642
2 Dawson-Hughes B, Harris SS, Krall EA, Dallal GE. Effect of calcium and vitamin D supplementation on bone density in men and women 65 years of age and older. N Engl J Med 1997; 337: 670–676

78 How to reduce the threatening risk of hip fractures in the elderly? Prophylactic therapy in old age?

Short answer: The risk of hip fracture can be reduced by early prevention or treatment of senile osteoporosis and by information and recommendations to reduce the risk of falling in the elderly.

Detailed answer: Spontaneous hip fractures are observed very rarely, e.g. the patients fall during walking due to the fracture. In most cases there is osteopenia or osteoporosis and a typical fall more or less involving the hip area is sufficient for fracturing. There are several possibilities to reduce the risk of hip fracture in the elderly population or in individual patients:

1. Early start of prevention of osteoporosis in men and women: assessment of risk factors, corresponding change in lifestyle, measurement of BMD, drug prevention in high risk cases.
2. In later life it is not too late: in patients with osteopenia calcium/vitamin D supplements may be sufficient as a first step. In patients with established osteoporosis specific antiosteoporotic medication.
3. Take history of potential risk factors for falling and give corresponding recommendations (see Question 79).
4. In persons with repeated falls in the past or in those having already suffered from one hip fracture a "hip protector" may be helpful (see Question 80).

79 Risk factors for falling and possibilities to counteract them

Short answer: The incidence of falls increases with age and falling is a very important contributing factor to hip and other non-vertebral fractures in the elderly.

It is very difficult to achieve a significant reduction in falls.

Detailed answer: Epidemiological studies show that 50% of women of age 85 will have one fall event per year. Not every fall is associated with a fracture. The complex pathogenesis of fracture events was discussed in Question 36 (see Fig. **4**). A large number of intrinsic and extrinsic risk factors has been identified which can be involved in numerous combinations in the individual fracture event (Table **20**).

From Table **20** it becomes obvious that it is very difficult to instruct elderly persons with the aim of reducing the incidence of falling. Indeed, the few studies that have been performed with this aim have

Table **20** Intrinsic and extrinsic risk factors for falls among the elderly

Intrinsic Risk Factors

1. Chronic illnesses: heart disease, Parkinson's and other neuromuscular disease, stroke, urinary incontinence, arthritis
2. Medications, alcohol: hypnotics, sedatives, antipsychotics, antidepressants, antiparkinson drugs, antihypertensives, alcohol
3. Sensory: vision, lower extremity sensory perception
4. Mental status: cognitive impairment, depression, dementia
5. Functional level: ADL, cane, walker use, history of falls
6. Gait, balance, strength: walking speed, postural sway, lower extremity strength, upper extremity strength, impaired reflexes

Extrinsic Risk Factors

1. Ground surface: throw rugs, loose carpets, slippery floors, cords and wires on floor, stairs with rugs or in poor repair
2. Furniture: clutter, unstable furniture, beds which are too high or too low, cabinets that are either too high or too low
3. Lighting: glare from unshielded windows or lamps, low or dim compounded by dark colored walls, absence of night lights
4. Bathroom: low toilet seat, no secure grab bars, absence of nonslip surfaces
5. Other: poorly maintained walking aids and equipment, improper shoes (not slip-resistant, high-heeled, too large).

shown very clearly that very complex and expensive intervention programs are necessary and the results are rather disappointing.

80 Is there new practical aid equipment and assistive devices?

Short answer: There is a large and increasing choice of excellent means of aid and assistive devices but they are too seldomly considered or used for the prevention of falls and fractures in the elderly.

Detailed answer: The large number of single or combined causative factors for falls in the elderly are shown in Table **20** (Question 79). The most frequent and important problems in advanced age are gait disturbances with reduced walking speed and impaired balance. Contributing factors include: fear of falling since previous fall, reduced muscle

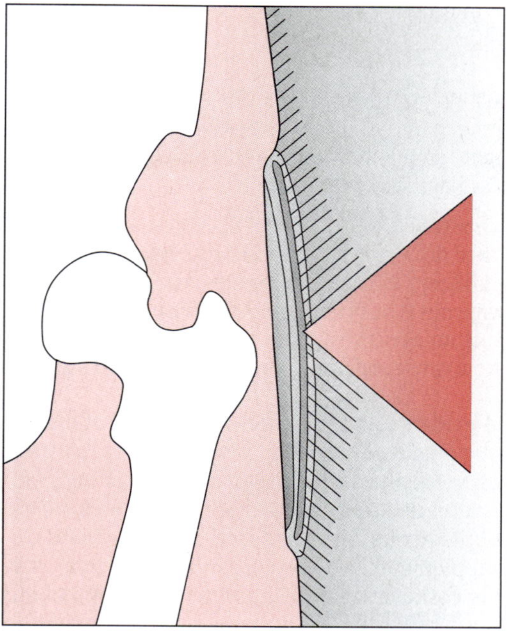

Fig. **10** Hip protector: The protector shield is anatomically designed to shunt the energy of an impact away from the greater trochanter to the surrounding soft tissue.

strength, impaired reflexes, neurological and/or rheumatological diseases. The possible aids include a simple cane or walking stick, crutches, walker (zimmer frame), or wheel chair. An important aid may be to raise the toilet seat, use a tub chair in the bathtub, etc.

A new simple and very effective device in this context is the "hip protector" (Fig. **10**).

Since in most cases of hip fracture the immediate cause of fracture is a sideways fall with direct impact on the greater trochanter it is a logical option to use a device to protect the hips, so that at the time of a fall the force and energy of the impact is attenuated and shunted away. A group from Finland has done a study on 1409 ambulatory but frail patients [1]. The relative risk in the hip protector group was 0.4, i.e. a 60% reduction in hip fractures could be demonstrated for this simple device.

Reference

1 Kannus P, Parkkari J, Niemi S, Pasanen M, Palvanen M, Jarvinen M, Vuori I. Prevention of hip fracture in elderly people with use of a hip protector. N Engl J Med 2000; 343: 1506 – 1513

81 Would it make sense to give calcium/vitamin D supplements to all elderly persons?

Short answer: Due to the high prevalence of insufficient calcium/vitamin D supply and the pathogenetic importance of the resulting secondary hyperparathyroidism, a general supplementation in the elderly could be advocated as a reasonable and economic concept.

Detailed answer: (See also Questions 77 and 78). Since health insurances in most countries are not very interested in prevention it may be difficult to institute the concept of a general prevention of fractures in the elderly by calcium/vitamin D substitution. Another problem would be the question of defining an age threshold.

Nevertheless, there are many good arguments favoring such a general health initiative:

1. There is accumulated evidence that insufficient calcium/vitamin D supply is extremely frequent in advanced age and plays an important role in the pathogenesis of senile osteoporosis and hip fracture risk.
2. A reduction of hip fractures and other non-vertebral fractures during calcium/vitamin D supplementation is evidence-based medicine.
3. Calcium/vitamin D supplements are very cheap and the total cost would be far below the costs for treatment and rehabilitation of hip fractures.
4. With the supplements used in low doses (e.g. 1000 mg calcium, 800 IU vitamin D) there are no risks or relevant adverse events.
5. It is not necessary to measure 25-OH-D by a rather expensive assay to prove D-deficiency. Low normal serum calcium (< 2.2 mmol/L), hypocalcuria, and slightly increased alkaline phosphatase are indicators for a deficit in calcium/vitamin D. A strong indicator are elevated levels of PTH.

Further information: R. Francis (Newcastle, UK) has shown in a nice study that alfacalcidol is superior to plain vitamin D in the management of osteoporosis.

Male Osteoporosis

82 Osteoporosis in men: onset, average age, practical management?

Short answer: Osteoporosis in men is observed from early childhood through advanced age. A thorough clinical assessment of stage, risk factors, and possible underlying diseases is mandatory as a basis for therapeutic decisions.

Detailed answer: The prevalence of osteoporosis in men was underestimated in the past. Today it is estimated that 10 – 20% of all patients with clinically relevant osteoporosis are men (see Question 4). In our prospective assessment of risk factors in 400 men with osteoporosis the age range was 12 – 88 years with a mean age of 55.6 years [1].

For practical management it is important to define the clinical stage of osteoporosis based on BMD and prevalent or missing fractures (see Table 7, Question 20). The second important point is to detect possible risk factors and/or underlying diseases to make a diagnosis of primary or secondary osteoporosis. In the above mentioned study [1], 52% had primary, 48% secondary osteoporosis. All existing studies show about 50% of secondary osteoporosis on average, that means a significantly higher percentage than in women.

In secondary osteoporosis there may be a chance to counteract the revealed risk factors or to treat the underlying diseases (e.g. hypogonadism, see Question 86). In the other cases and in primary osteoporosis the same therapeutic agents as in women can be used (except estrogen and raloxifen). For most of these drugs, however, there are no data available that have been generated in sufficiently large studies.

Reference

1 Ringe JD, Dorst AJ, Faber H. Osteoporosis in men – Clinical assessment of 400 patients and 205 controls by risk factor analysis, densitometry, and X-ray findings. Osteologie 1997; 6: 81 – 86

83 Assessment of osteoporosis in men: screening for which risk factors ?

Short answer: The most important and frequent risk factors are long-term corticoid therapy, hypogonadism, hypercalcuria, heavy nicotine and alcohol consumption. Numerous further single or combined risk factors can be found by careful investigation.

Detailed answer: The pattern of risk factors to be found in men with osteoporosis varies in different studies according to the specialization of the respective investigating centers. A large number of male patients were referred to our department of general internal medicine (with specialization for bone disease) during the last years for investigation of suspected osteoporosis, i.e. it was not a selection of mainly endocrinological cases as in several other studies [1]. They were mainly sent by general practitioners and orthopedists, i.e. the mixture of revealed risk factors reflects the male population with back pain and/or vertebral fractures.

From these we have screened 400 men referred consecutively to our department with a standardized program for clinical investigation and identified the 26 different risk factors shown in Table **21** (listed in order of decreasing prevalence).

Reference

1 Ringe JD, Dorst AJ, Faber H. Osteoporosis in men – Clinical assessment of 400 patients and 205 controls by risk factor analysis, densitometry, and X-ray findings. Osteologie 1997; 6: 81–86

84 Are there accepted strategies for prevention of osteoporosis in men?

Short answer: Population-based strategies and individually adapted measures can be used for prevention. For the latter, identification of possible risk factors is a prerequisite.

Detailed answer: In men, too, inactivity, long-term poor calcium diet, a phosphate- and/or protein-rich nutrition, alcohol, and smoking are changeable risk factors for a low bone mass and high fracture risk. These risk factors should be reduced in the general population.

For individual prevention the following recommendations can be given [1]:

- Bone densitometry should be performed in men with risk factors (see Table **21**), osteoporosis in the family, chronic back pain, and prevalent low-trauma fractures.

Table **21** Type and frequency of risk factors found in 400 consecutive cases of male osteoporosis [1]

Risk factor	n	(%)	Risk factor	n	(%)
Heavy smoking	96	24.0	Hyperthyroidism	9	2.4
High alcohol consumption	87	21.8	Diabetes mellitus	9	2.3
Long-term corticoids	72	18.0	Multiple myeloma	8	2.0
Hypophosphatemia	44	11.0	Lymphoproliferative disease	5	1.3
Hypercalcuria (poss. plus kidney stones)	37	9.3	Thyroxin therapy	5	1.3
Hypogonadism	35	8.8	Heparin therapy	4	1.0
Liver disease	24	6.0	Primary hyperparathyroidism	4	1.0
Crohn's disease	24	6.0	Bone marrow carcinosis	2	0.5
Calcium deficiency	24	6.0	Osteogenesis imperfecta	1	0.3
Chronic obstructive lung disease	23	5.8	Systemic mastocytosis	1	0.3
Gastric surgery	16	4.0	Cushing's disease	1	0.3
Physical inactivity, immobility	15	3.8	Rheumatoid arthritis	1	0.3
Anticonvulsants	12	3.0	Mild renal insufficiency	1	0.3

- In patients with low-normal BMD values, a "healthy-for-bone" nutrition and a regular training program should be started.
- Patients with osteopenia (preclinical osteoporosis) should be further investigated. Detected risk factors should be eliminated as far as possible and underlying diseases should be treated.
- In elderly men the strategies for hip fracture prevention are the same as in women: calcium/vitamin D, prevent falls, in selected cases hip protector.

Reference

1 Hosking D, Ringe J. (Eds). Treatment of metabolic bone disease. Management strategy and drug therapy. Martin Dunitz, London, 2000

85 Bisphosphonates in established osteoporosis in men ?

Short answer: Recent studies show that the therapeutic results obtained with bisphosphonates are very similar in men and women with osteoporosis. Alendronate is the first bisphosphonate that received the label effective in the treatment of osteoporosis in men.

Detailed answer: In a multicenter study performed in the USA and Europe, 241 men with osteoporosis (30% with low testosterone) were treated for 2 years with 10 mg/day alendronate [1]. The effect on BMD at the lumbar spine and proximal femur and on the markers of bone turnover were very consistent with the well known average changes observed in postmenopausal osteoporosis and the number of patients with new vertebral fractures was lower in the alendronate than in the placebo group.

Our independent, controlled 2-year study of 134 men with primary osteoporosis confirmed the positive effects of this bisphosphonate on BMD and fracture incidence.

We assume that etidronate, risedronate, and ibandronate given to osteoporotic men in adequate doses will similarly result in positive therapeutic effects as known from trials in postmenopausal women.

Reference

1 Orwoll E, Ettinger M, Weiss S, Miller P, Kendler D, Graham J, Adami S, Weber K, Lorenc R, Pietschmann P, Vandormael K, Lombardi A. Alendronate for the treatment of osteoporosis in men. N Engl J Med 2000; 343: 604–610

86 Is hormone replacement with testosterone a reasonable therapeutic option in men with osteoporosis?

Short answer: A general hormone substitution with androgens to prevent osteoporosis in men is not justified. In men with hypogonadism (proven testosterone deficiency), however, several small studies have documented increments in BMD.

Detailed answer: In patients with the clinical symptoms of hypogonadism and significantly lowered free testosterone levels, androgen treatment can be recommended for prevention and treatment of osteoporosis, e.g. 250 mg testosterone *i.m.* every 2 – 3 weeks. With oral testosterone administration to reach sufficient plasma levels is difficult. A new modality for administration is transdermal testosterone. Patches are available which deliver 2.5 mg per 24 hours and the resulting plasma levels are sufficiently stable.

Further information: In the United Kingdom an androgen study was performed in eugonadal men with primary osteoporosis. It was shown in that particular trial that androgens were transformed in part to estrogen and that the increased rates in BMD correlated better with serum estrogen than with testosterone levels. The authors have not observed negative effects on the pattern of lipoproteins or any significant increase in PSA levels.

87 Should fluoride be used in male osteoporosis?

Short answer: There are no placebo-controlled studies with fluoride in established male osteoporosis with prevalent fractures. In our study of men with stage 1 osteoporosis without prevalent vertebral fractures we found favorable effects with a rather low dose intermittent monofluorophosphate (MFP)/calcium regimen.

Detailed answer: In numerous older trials studying the effect of fluoride in osteoporosis some male cases were included. The results always showed that the response to fluoride in terms of increasing BMD values is not different between men and women.

The so far largest study including only men was done prospectively in 60 men. Inclusion criteria were primary osteoporosis, lumbar spine BMD < – 2.5 SD and no prevalent vertebral fractures. The patients received 114 mg MFP per day (= 15 mg fluoride ions) with an intermittent 3 months on, 1 month off regimen. After three years we found an average increase of 8.9% at the spine, 1.9% at the femoral neck, and 7.7% at the distal radius. During the time of observation the percentage of patients suffering from first vertebral fractures was significantly lower in the MFP/Ca group than in the group with calcium monotherapy [1].

These encouraging data have not been confirmed by other studies up to now, i.e. the evidence is not sufficient to recommend fluoride as a treatment in early osteoporosis in men.

In a small pilot study on 15 male patients recruited according to the same diagnostic criteria, we found significantly higher increments of BMD when combining MFP/Ca with alfacalcidol (Table **22**).

Table **22** Effects of a low-dose intermittent fluoride/calcium regimen alone or combined with 1 µg alfacalcidol on lumbar spine and femoral neck BMD in men with primary osteoporosis stage 1

Average changes of BMD after 3 years of therapy			
	Intermittent MFP/Ca	Continuous Ca	Intermittent MFP/Ca plus alfacalcidol
n	30	30	15
L2 – L4	+ 8.9%	– 2.4%	+ 15.6%
Femoral neck	+ 1.9%	– 1.4%	+ 4.8%

Reference

1 Ringe JD, Dorst A, Kipshoven C, Rovati LC, Setnikar I. Avoidance of vertebral fractures in men with idiopathic osteoporosis by a three year therapy with calcium and low-dose intermittent monofluorophosphate. Osteoporosis Int 1998; 8: 47 – 52

Secondary and Localized Forms of Osteoporosis

88 What is the definition of secondary osteoporosis?

Short answer: The diagnosis of secondary osteoporosis is made in patients in whom the development of bone loss can be clearly attributed to a disease, drug therapy, or a combination of relevant risk factors.

Detailed answer: During diagnostic assessment of patients with osteoporosis the rate of secondary cases will increase with the intensity of investigation. Accordingly, the number of cases of secondary osteoporosis is much higher in men than in postmenopausal women because, as a matter of fact, physicians tend to investigate more carefully in men.

The first and most important diagnostic step is a thorough history of possible risk factors, medications, and underlying diseases known to have negative effects on calcium and bone metabolism.

A distinction should be made between monoetiological secondary osteoporosis where one distinct risk factor, disease, or medication is the clear single cause of osteoporosis and, on the other hand, polyetiological forms where several factors contribute to the negative bone balance and the development of osteoporosis. Again, the more detailed the history and the more corresponding laboratory tests are extended, the more likely it is that several risk factors or an overlap of different factors will be detected (Fig. **11**).

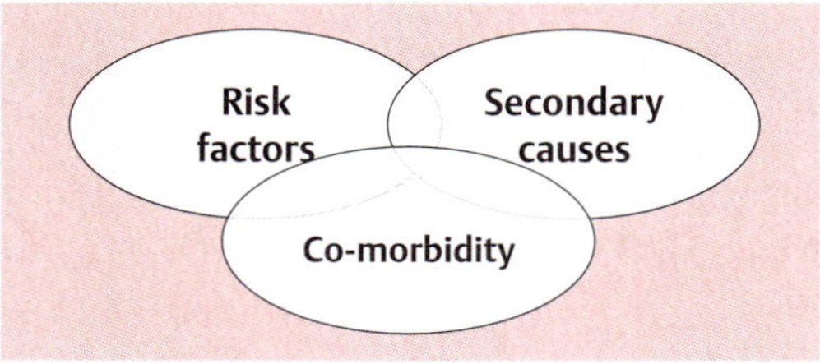

Fig. **11** Definition of secondary osteoporosis?

The numerous risk factors/diseases that we identified in 400 men are shown in Table **20** (see Question 83).

One of the problems in diagnosing secondary osteoporosis is that there are no clear thresholds for several risk factors. For example it is up to the examining physician to make a decision about what amount of alcohol drinking for what period of time, what intensity of smoking, and what degree of inactivity or low calcium intake should be considered a risk.

Even for corticoid-induced osteoporosis, no clear threshold dose or duration of use has been defined (see Question 90).

89 Is primary hyperparathyroidism a risk factor for secondary osteoporosis?

Short answer: A long-term undetected and untreated primary hyperparathyroidism very frequently leads to kidney stones but also to bone loss and fractures. After surgical correction of the endocrinological disease, a persisting secondary osteoporosis may require medical treatment.

Detailed answer: The highly increased bone turnover due to permanently increased PTH secretion can lead to a severe bone disease with generalized bone loss, development of multiple cystic lesions, and subperiosteal erosions histologically known as "osteitis fibrosa generalisata" (von Recklinghausen).

After surgical removal of the parathyroid adenoma, mild forms of osteopenia may heal spontaneously but in more advanced forms an inactive secondary osteoporosis may persist (histologically not different from osteoporosis).

These patients have a significantly increased fracture risk and very often the spontaneous repair of bone substance after operations is insufficient. In patients with T score values < – 3.0 after operation or with insufficient increase one year later a drug treatment for osteoporosis should be started. In mild cases calcium or Ca/D can be tried as a first step, in more severe cases HRT, raloxifen, alfacalcidol, or bisphosphonates may be considered.

90 What dose and duration of oral corticoid therapy induces a significant risk of osteoporosis?

Short answer: A threshold dose and duration of oral corticosteroids for the development of osteoporosis has not been defined. The clinical manifestation of osteoporosis often depends on different cofactors, e.g. underlying disease, comedication, and further risk factors.

Detailed answer: In the literature threshold values for oral corticoids between 5 and 15 mg/day have been described. Doses below 7.5 mg are very often cited as being relatively harmless. There is, however, no scientific support for this assumption. From more recent data it can be concluded that long-term low-dose treatment with doses of 2.5 – 5 mg prednisolone per day will lead to corticoid-induced osteoporosis (CIO).

In several studies a rough correlation between the cumulative dose of oral corticoids and BMD was found. Alternate day administration does not reduce the risk of CIO. Topical application of corticoids has a lower risk but it has been shown very recently that even with inhaled corticoids there is a significant risk of CIO.

Concerning the duration of corticoid therapy there are data supporting the view that the highest rates of bone loss will occur during the first half year. In most cases this is also the time of relatively higher doses and only thereafter are lower maintenance doses given. A three months treatment with a rather high dosage may already be detrimental for the bone.

Further information: The main problem in this context is in fact that in most patients BMD is not measured at the onset of a long-term corticoid therapy. That means the physician in charge has no idea whether the patient has a rather good BMD or already suffers from osteopenia when starting with corticoid medication. We recommend carrying out BMD determination in every patient starting long-term corticoid therapy.

91 Are there safe means to prevent the development of osteoporosis during ongoing corticoid medication?

Short answer: Today we have a choice of very effective substances which are able to delay or even to avoid osteoporosis during corticoid medication, when started early and used correctly.

Detailed answer: It is estimated that in most countries only 10% of the patients on long-term corticosteroid medication receive simultaneously an "osteoprotective" medication, i.e. in 90% of the cases physicians miss the chance of early prevention. As a consequence we see new patients every day with established corticosteroid-induced osteoporosis (CIO) presenting with significant osteopenia, back pain, and fractures.

In most cases the pathogenesis of CIO is complex: besides corticoid medication contributing factors are, e.g. the underlying disease, inactivity, muscle wasting, other medications.

Evaluation of co-risk-factors and results of initial BMD determination are decisive for the preventive measures. According to the BMD results and individual risk factors the following recommendations can be given:

- *Normal or high BMD (T score + 2.0 to − 1.0), without additional risk factors:* High calcium diet, program of gymnastics, possibly low dose calcium/vitamin D supplementation.
- *Osteopenia (T score − 1.0 to − 2.5), plus additional risk factors:* Calcium/vitamin D supplement; in postmenopausal women HRT; alternatively and in men: calcitonin nasal spray, alfacalcidol 1 µg/day, alendronate 5 mg, risedronate 2.5 mg.
- *Established osteoporosis (T score < − 2.5),with or without fractures and further risk factors:* Bisphosphonates orally or *i.v.* plus Ca/D; alfacalcidol 1 µg + 500 mg calcium (poss. combinations with HRT, raloxifen).

92 Is vitamin D contraindicated in sarcoidosis treated with corticosteroids?

Short answer: Serum calcium should be measured. In patients with high normal or elevated levels no plain vitamin D or vitamin D analogue should be given for the prevention of corticosteroid-induced osteoporosis (CIO).

Detailed answer: Hypercalcemia is a well known complication of sarcoidosis observed in about 10 – 15% of patients. An adequate corticoid therapy reduces the risk of this complication. The underlying mechanism is an augmented extrarenal 1-hydroxylation of 25-hydroxycholecalciferol in the sarcoid granulomata. This phenomenon of extrarenal vitamin D activation is also observed in other granulomatous diseases (tuberculosis, berylliosis, granulomas after silicone implants, etc.).

Since calcium/vitamin D is important as a first-step measure in the fight against CIO we do not advocate a complete renunciation of this therapeutic option. The same is true for alfacalcidol, which may have a lower risk than plain vitamin D because it is already 1-hydroxylated.

The following practical recommendations can be given:

- Serum calcium levels should be in the normal range.
- If calcium is in the high-normal range (2.50 – 2.65 mmol/L) start calcium/vitamin D with low doses (400 IU vitamin D, 500 mg calcium).
- Control serum calcium after 2 – 3 weeks and at individually adapted intervals thereafter.

Attention: In patients with sarcoidosis, hypercalcemia may become apparent after intense exposure to sunlight (= increased production of cholecalciferol in the skin), i.e. season and sun exposure of the patient have to be taken into consideration.

93 Therapeutic results with alfacalcidol in corticoid-induced osteoporosis (CIO) ?

Short answer: Due to its therapeutic profile alfacalcidol is of special interest in this condition. Several sufficiently extensive studies have shown that alfacalcidol is a well tolerated and effective drug in the fight against CIO and is superior to plain vitamin D.

Detailed answer: A recent review of the literature on prevention of CIO showed clearly that in most cases calcium plus plain vitamin D is not sufficient to avoid further bone loss. This supplementation has only small effects in patients with unequivocal vitamin D deficiency during the first few months of administration [1].

The D-analogue alfacalcidol bypasses the feed-back controlled activation in the kidney, i.e. is an active hormonal treatment and not a nutritional substitution (see Question 57).

Several trials studying the efficacy of alfacalcidol in CIO (Verstraeten et al. 1989, Lakatos et al. 1996, Reginster et al. 1999) demonstrated positive effects in prevention and therapy. We directly compared [1] the effects of plain vitamin D (1000 IU + 500 mg calcium) and alfacalcidol (1 µg + 500 mg calcium) in 124 patients with established CIO and found highly significant differences in the second and third year of treatment (Fig. **12**).

Reference

1 Ringe JD, Faber H. Calcium and vitamin D in the prevention and treatment of glucocorticoid-induced osteoporosis. Clin Exp Rheumatol 2000; 18 Suppl 21: S44 – S48

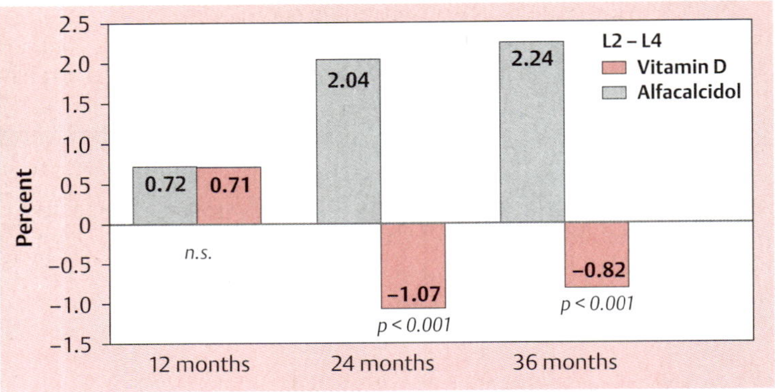

Fig. **12** Mean changes in BMD at the lumbar spine (% of initial values) during a 3-year period of treatment with an active D-analog + calcium or plain vitamin D + calcium in 124 patients on long-term corticoid therapy.

94 Prevention and treatment of corticoid-induced osteoporosis (CIO) in children and adolescents?

Short answer: Use primarily all options of "basic treatment" (see Question 45). In severe cases introduce pharmacological therapy – as far as possible with "physiological substances" that are not deposited in bone tissue.

Detailed answer:

Prevention of CIO in children and adolescents:

1. Calcium-rich diet, daily program of gymnastics, reduction of corticoids as low as possible. Calcium/vitamin D supplementation adapted to age and body weight.
2. Second control of BMD 6 – 12 months after start of corticoids. If BMD decreases significantly despite basic measures start treatment with, e.g. nasal calcitonin 200 IU/day or alfacalcidol 1 µg/day.

Therapy for established CIO in children and adolescents:

1. In cases with significantly lowered BMD with or without fractures start with basic treatment (see above) and combine with "physiological drugs" (e.g. calcitonin, alfacalcidol, see above).
2. In severe, treatment-resistant cases bisphophonates may be indicated with oral or intravenous administration. First communications on single cases reported positive effects. There is, however, no experience with the long-term consequences of bisphosphonate deposition in the growing skeleton. Therefore, this treatment should be restricted to very severe and desperate cases.

95 Should children receive calcium supplements to prevent osteoporosis in later life?

Short answer: A regular and optimal calcium supply during childhood by nutrition or supplements favors skeletal development and the amount of peak bone mass in young adulthood.

Detailed answer: In several epidemiological studies a positive correlation between average calcium uptake and bone mass was shown for children. Since milk and dairy products are the nutrients that offer the by far the highest calcium supply, alimentation of children should contain a high proportion of milk and milk products.

The consumption of soft drinks like "Coca Cola" may be detrimental due to the rather high phosphate contents inhibiting intestinal calcium absorption.

The recommended daily calcium supply for children is 500 – 1000 mg calcium. There is no risk with higher amounts since the enteric resorption is limited to 20 – 30%. The surplus calcium will be excreted without problems in the feces.

In children with lactase deficiency or proven milk-protein intolerance, regular calcium supplements are mandatory to compensate for the missing intake of dairy products.

96 What are the possibilities to avoid severe immobility-induced osteoporosis after transverse lesion of the cord with paraplegia?

Short answer: The acute and dramatic process of bone resorption after spinal cord injury can be delayed or stopped by a potent antiresorptive therapy.

Detailed answer: The systemic secondary osteoporosis developing very rapidly after high spinal cord injury is a very impressive and sad model for acute osteoporosis of immobilization. In spite of the quite large numbers of persons suffering from this type of injury every year, there are only few prospective densitometric and even fewer intervention studies.

BMD measurements performed on immobilized healthy young men by the NASA showed BMD losses at the calcaneus of 30 – 40% within a few weeks. More recent results from cosmonauts of the Russian Mir space station showed a significant loss of bone and lean tissue during long duration space flights in spite of the current in-flight exercise program [1].

The same has been shown for patients with paraplegia. The main loss of bone mass occurs during the first 6 months after spinal cord injury. There is an increased risk of kidney stones during this period due to high bone resorption.

Nearly 20 years ago Minaire from St Etienne was able to show that the rapid bone loss in these patients can be stopped by daily injections of 100 IU salmon calcitonin [2].

No large studies with bisphosphonates have been published so far. We suggest that especially an initial *i.v.* therapy with bisphosphonates could prove to be very effective.

Since patients with spinal cord lesions have a rather high life expectancy today and since fractures lead to significant morbidity, the necessity of preventing osteoporosis is obvious.

References

1 LeBlanc A, Schneider V, Shackelford L, West S, Organov V, Bakulin A, Voronin L. Bone mineral and lean tissue loss after long duration space flight. J Musculoskel Neuron Interact 2000; 1: 157 – 160

2 Minaire P, Depassio J, Meunier P, Edouard C, Caulin F, Pilochery G, Julien DA. Treatment of active osteoporosis due to paraplegia with calcitonin. Calcif Tiss Int 1983; Suppl. 35, 259

97 Secondary osteoporosis due to thyroxin therapy: what can we do?

Short answer: Negative effects on the skeleton can be avoided by early diagnosis and treatment of hyperthyroidism (Graves' disease) and avoidance of too high doses of thyroxin when substitution is indicated.

Detailed answer: Thyroxin induces an increased bone turnover. An undetected endogenous overproduction or long-term use of high doses of this hormone may lead to secondary osteoporosis. Secondary osteoporosis due only to this mechanism is, however, observed very rarely today.

A long-term moderate overdosage of thyroxin may be a contributing risk factor in patients with polyetiological secondary osteoporosis. The impact of the thyroxin treatment on the development of osteoporosis remains unclear in most cases. Since postmenopausal women very often have osteopenia (preclinical osteoporosis), Graves' disease or inadequate thyroxin treatment may in some cases be the trigger for established disease. In such patients BMD should be measured, endogenous or exogenous thyroxin should be reduced, and treatment of osteoporosis should be started.

Patients with previous carcinoma of the thyroid receiving high, suppressive doses of thyroxin mostly have a significantly increased risk of osteoporosis.

98 Are there new therapeutic concepts for osteogenesis imperfecta (OI)?

Short answer: OI is a heterogeneous group of disorders principally affecting type I collagen and leading to increased bone fragility. Recently, cyclic intravenous treatment with pamidronate has been proved to be beneficial for children with severe forms of OI.

Detailed answer: OI, often referred to as "brittle bone disease", is a hereditary disorder that is characterized by either qualitative or quantitative abnormalities in type I collagen. OI can be classified into four major types according to clinical, radiographic, and genetic criteria.

Numerous therapeutic agents such as sodium fluoride, magnesium oxide, anabolic steroids, and ascorbic acid have been shown to be not consistently effective. A Japanese group showed a positive trend on fractures with intranasal administration of calcitonin. Positive effects with human growth hormone (hGH) have also been reported.

The most promising treatment for children and adults with this severe debilitating bone disease today is bisphosphonate therapy. Bone marrow transplants remain an interesting experimental option.

Glorieux et al. treated 30 children with severe OI (age range 3 – 16 years) with cyclic pamidronate infusions in an uncontrolled observational study [1]. They found a reduction in bone resorption, increases in bone density, and improved clinical outcomes.

We have done a pilot study in 12 adults with moderate to severe OI using a combined intermittent treatment regimen of etidronate, fluoride, calcium and vitamin D (EFCaD) and found very impressive increases in lumbar spine and femoral neck BMD.

A controlled trial with bisphosphonates might establish the exact role of these drugs in this debilitating disease.

Reference

1 Glorieux FH, Bishop NJ, Plotkin H, Chabot G, Lanoue G, Travers R. Cyclical administration of pamidronate in children with severe osteogenesis imperfecta. N Engl J Med 1998; 339: 947 – 952

99 What is the therapeutic value of calcitonin in algodystrophy (reflex sympathetic dystrophy syndrome, Sudeck's syndrome)?

Short answer: With daily subcutaneous injections of 100 IU of salmon calcitonin very often an early decrease in pain and later remineralization and functional improvement can be achieved.

Detailed answer: Algodystrophy is a rather frequent complication in traumatology with often significant functional impairment of the affected limb. Typical symptoms are severe local pain, dystrophic changes of skin and bone, and impaired strength and mobility.

Physiotherapy, treatment with NSAIDs, injections of novocain into the sympathetic ganglia, and glucocorticoids have been used in the past with little success.

The introduction of calcitonin treatment was a breakthrough in algodystrophy therapy. The very positive effects were explained by the specific inhibition of osteoclasts together with the analgesic potency of calcitonin and vascular effects (vasodilation). The best results will be obtained with early diagnosis and very early start of calcitonin injections. In the later stages of algodystrophy the rate of non-responders increases.

In recent years, bisphosphonates with oral or intravenous administration have been tried in patients with algodystrophy. Some authors reported even better results than with the classical calcitonin therapy. Controlled studies with bisphosphonates are still lacking.

100 What is the current recommended treatment for transient osteoporosis of the hip?

Short answer: Although this rare localized form of osteoporosis mostly ends with spontaneous remission, bisphosphonate treatment can be recommended to accelerate pain relief and healing.

Detailed answer: Transient, circumscribed osteoporosis affects mainly the hip (proximal femur). Other rare manifestations can be found in the knee or foot region. Etiology and pathogenesis have not yet been elucidated. Mechanisms similar to the reflex sympathetic dystrophy syndrome (Question 99) are discussed. But, in general, there is no previous trauma or operation at the affected site. Rather frequently, transient osteoporosis of the hip is associated with pregnancy.

The most relevant diagnostic procedure is magnetic resonance imaging (MRI). MR images show increased joint fluid and diffuse signal abnormalities in the bone marrow of the affected femoral head and/or neck.

The treatment strategy comprises analgesic/anti-inflammatory therapy with NSAIDs, walking aids, and bisphosphonates. Based on our clinical experience with several cases during recent years, we recommend infusions of 60 mg pamidronate or 4 mg ibandronate. In most cases, pain relief and functional improvement will be reached within a few weeks.

Index

E

F

H

I

K

L

M

N

O

P

Q

R

S

T

U

V

X

DATE DUE